The Iconic Power of the Short Story

The Iconic Power of the Short Story

Exploring Culture, Cognition, and Affective Involvement in Seamus Heaney

Carmen M. Bretones Callejas

PETER LANG
Oxford - Berlin - Bruxelles - Chennai - Lausanne - New York

Bibliographic information published by the Deutsche Nationalbibliothek. The German National Library lists this publication in the German National Bibliography; detailed bibliographic data is available on the Internet at http://dnb.d-nb.de.

A catalogue record for this book is available from the British Library.

Library of Congress Cataloging-in-Publication Data

Names: Bretones, Carmen M., author.
Title: The iconic power of the short story : exploring culture, cognition, and affective involvement in Seamus Heaney / Carmen M. Bretones Callejas.
Description: Oxford ; New York : Peter Lang, [2024] | Includes bibliographical references and index.
Identifiers: LCCN 2024047616 (print) | LCCN 2024047617 (ebook) | ISBN 9781803744322 (paperback) | ISBN 9781803744339 (ebook) | ISBN 9781803744346 (epub)
Subjects: LCSH: Heaney, Seamus, 1939-2013—Criticism and interpretation. | Heaney, Seamus, 1939-2013—Literary style. | Short story. | English poetry—Irish authors—History and criticism.
Classification: LCC PR6058.E2 Z558 2024 (print) | LCC PR6058.E2 (ebook) | DDC 821/.914—dc23/eng/20241127
LC record available at https://lccn.loc.gov/2024047616
LC ebook record available at https://lccn.loc.gov/2024047617

Cover illustration by Carmen M. Bretones Callejas
Cover design by Peter Lang Group AG

ISBN 978-1-80374-432-2 (print)
ISBN 978-1-80374-433-9 (ePDF)
ISBN 978-1-80374-434-6 (ePub)
DOI 10.3726/b21631

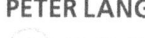 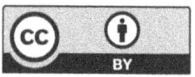

Open Access: This work is licensed under a Creative Commons Attribution CC-BY 4.0 license. To view a copy of this license, visit https://creativecommons.org/licenses/by/4.0/

© 2024 Carmen M. Bretones Callejas
Published by Peter Lang Ltd, Oxford, United Kingdom
info@peterlang.com – www.peterlang.com

Carmen M. Bretones Callejas has asserted her right under the Copyright, Designs and Patents Act, 1988, to be identified as Author of this Work.

This publication has been peer reviewed.

Contents

List of Figures — vii

The Cognitive Power of Story: A Foreword by Mark Turner — ix

Preface — xiii

Acknowledgments — xv

CHAPTER 1
Introduction — 1

CHAPTER 2
The Subject — 5

CHAPTER 3
The Iconic Power of the Short Story — 41

CHAPTER 4
Story, Metaphor and the Cognitive Phenomenon — 65

CHAPTER 5
Textual Analysis — 81

CHAPTER 6
Conclusions — 113

Bibliography — 117

Annex — 127

Figures

Figure 1.	Important geographical locations in Heaney's Ireland	17
Figure 2.	Basic diagram representing the process of blending	23
Figure 3.	Metaphorical patterns that show how "anger" is conceptualized	31
Figure 4.	Primary metaphors in English	32
Figure 5.	General model of metaphorical transfers among sensory modalities	78
Figure 6.	Model of metaphorical transfers among sensory modalities in the poetry of Seamus Heaney	78
Figure 7.	Integrated Textual Analysis Model	85

The Cognitive Power of Story: A Foreword by Mark Turner

Story is a basic principle of mind. Most of our experience, our knowledge, and our thinking is organized as stories. Human language itself depends upon our advanced ability to think in stories. Given the fundamental cognitive role of story, it is of course to be found everywhere in human cognition; it is not at all restricted to prose or even writing. It is used by poets, politicians, and artists of all kinds to guide us to tight and coherent conceptions of otherwise diffuse and intractable conceptual networks, whose many, often unintegrated streams of meaning need some cognitive condensation, some iconic unity, if they are to stick in the mind. The short story, as a literary form, is revered for its power to guide the reader to concise and memorable compressions of resonant emotional, intellectual, and cultural complexities. Cognitive scientists often turn to short stories as a kind of laboratory specimen for investigating how human beings construct and seize upon meaning.

The Iconic Power of the Short Story explores the cognitive processes of story by showing how Seamus Heaney, a great and influential poet, uses them. Heaney's characteristic narrative technique offers a marvelous lens on the workings of the mind. The mind is embodied and affective; it operates in cultural contexts, often through action, and it exploits whatever it can find or build in its environments to aid its thinking. What it can find and build includes other people. The Iconic Power of the Short Story shows us Heaney at work to use story under conditions of embodiment and affect, context and culture. Bretones Callejas guides us through the nuanced landscapes of Heaney's poetry, examining the cognitive mechanisms that give poetry its iconic power.

The mental scope of story is magnified by various kinds of conceptual projection and integration—one story can help us grasp another. Different stories can be blended into a tight compression, and basic connections can come to be entrenched as metaphors. These entrenched connections are always ripe for further exploration and refinement, beginning within their original conceptual integration networks. Heaney routinely conducts such refinements and explorations. As Bretones Callejas shows, Heaney's use of projection, metaphor, and blending is far from decorative; instead, Heaney uses them as powerful cognitive tools for constructing meaning, and especially for forging connections between the familiar and the unknown.

Although the advanced powers of the human mind for story, projection, compression, and blending are species-wide, available to all cognitively modern human beings, they are only tools, not products. It can require a long time and great distributed work to use these tools to create specific cultural products. These cognitive tools make it possible for human beings to be so creative, to produce impressive ranges of art, music, fashion, dress, grammar, language, poetry, mathematical insight, scientific discovery, advanced tool conception, advanced social cognition, and so on. They are what makes culture possible. Different groups of human beings use them to create somewhat different conceptual products and different cultures, and those cultural arrays are in turn inputs to the underlying cognitive operations of story and projection. Heaney's poetry showcases the way in which existing cultural products of cognition feed new work by the very cognitive operations that gave them rise. The result of this new cognitive work is new poems, conveying new conceptions. For Heaney, the landscape, history, and social dynamics of Northern Ireland provide cultural inputs to these new conceptions. Heaney specializes in exploring the pullulation and interaction between established cultural products of cognition and new cognitive work that results in new and extended meaning, delivering poems of muscular cognitive work, universal themes, and specific cultural settings. This characteristic dynamism of Heaney's work—new cognition on established cultural products, producing refinements—is a focal point of the book. Culture is both old and new: it is an output of previous creative cognition that serves as input to new cognitive work and, consequently, new cultural considerations.

The Iconic Power of the Short Story shows that impressive, even brilliant, practices of intuitive close reading can be made scientific and persuasive through the methods of cognitive science, especially cognitive linguistics, and specifically through lexical research and corpus linguistics.

The Cognitive Power of Story: A Foreword by Mark Turner xi

Bretones Callejas is a master of both the humanistic and the scientific approach; indeed, she shows implicitly that research on literature cannot profitably separate them. The result is, for the Heaney specialist, a series of detailed textual analyzes of Heaney's poems. But for everyone else, the result is a brilliant exploration of how specific, advanced human cognitive operations makes the power of poetry possible.

Preface

In the patchwork of time, where lives and stories intertwine, the paths we tread often intersect with the legacies of remarkable individuals. Born on April 13, 1973, my journey found resonance with the unfolding narrative of Seamus Heaney, a towering figure in the realm of literature. As I embarked on a year of exploration in 1995, my footsteps traced the landscapes of Northern Ireland as an Erasmus student exchanged from the University of Granada, Spain, to the University of Ulster at Coleraine. Little did I know that during that very year, the Nobel Prize in Literature would be bestowed upon Seamus Heaney, a poet of immense lyrical beauty and ethical depth. Also born on April 13, but some years before, 1939, in Castledawson, Northern Ireland, Heaney's words resonated in me and would resonate across time and space, speaking to the essence of everyday miracles and the living past.

Three years later, I met Helen Vendler, Heaney's friend and colleague at Harvard. I was a visiting doctoral researcher with Mark Turner at the University of Maryland at College Park, as well as visiting Joe Grady at Georgetown University, and she was invited to the department. Then I sensed that even though my core studies had to do with Language and Cognition, and I was visiting George Lakoff and Chuck Fillmore at the University of California at Berkeley with another grant soon, Heaney would always come across my path, and I decided to use his work as corpus of analysis for my thesis.

Some years later, in 2013, there was another touching parallel. A new chapter of my life unfolded when my beloved daughter came to this world, and unexpectedly Seamus Heaney's earthly journey came to an end. His death reverberated not just in me, but through literary and cultural communities, immortalizing him as one of the most celebrated poets of the twentieth and twenty-first centuries. The deep cultural and emotional connections that his works evoke, and his language as a cradle through which he mirrored and explored the depths of human experience, continue to inspire, and bridge gaps between different generations, fields of investigation, and lives.

Acknowledgments

I am deeply grateful to my research groups at the University of Almería, Language and Thought: Relationships of Meaning in Lexicon and Literary Works (HUM602) and Lidisfarne (HUM807), for their invaluable support and collaboration. Their insights and dedication have significantly enriched this work.

Special thanks are due to Mark Turner from Case Western Reserve University, whose profound expertise and thoughtful guidance have been a cornerstone in the development of this book. His generous gift of time and advice has been instrumental.

I am also indebted to Juani Guerra from the University of Las Palmas, whose wisdom and encouragement have been a source of inspiration throughout this journey. Her constant support has been deeply appreciated.

Bernard McGuirk form the University of Nottingham deserves heartfelt thanks for his critical insights and constructive feedback, which have greatly enhanced the quality of this book.

To my family, your endless patience, love, and support have been my anchor. Without your understanding and encouragement, this book would not have been possible. Thank you for always believing in me and giving me the strength to persevere.

To all, your contributions have been immeasurable, and I am profoundly thankful for the privilege of working with such esteemed and supportive colleagues, as well as for the unwavering support of my family.

CHAPTER 1

Introduction

In the realm of literary exploration, *the short story* stands as a form of expression that encapsulates profound narratives within concise confines (Lohafer, 2003, May, 2013). As we explore the domain of the short story, we reveal a world where the literary mind finds its reflection and where the art of storytelling becomes the materialization of the cognitive processes that shape our understanding of the world and our place within it (see Turner, 1996; Lakoff and Johnson, 1999; Gibbs, 1994; Brosch, 2014, 2017; Herman, 2007). One luminary who shows the literary craft with virtuosity is Seamus Heaney, an acclaimed wordsmith whose works radiate an iconic power that resonates deeply. As we venture on a journey through Heaney's works, we approach a tapestry interwoven with cultural insights, cognitive elements, and emotive engagement, illuminating the magnitude of his storytelling power and its capacity to forge profound connections with readers in surprising ways.

Central to the dynamic interplay of mind and imagination lies the short story—a compact yet profoundly expressive vehicle of narrative that encapsulates the very rhythms and constructs of thought itself. Much like the mind's inclination for transforming complex ideas into succinct forms, the short story stands as a basic transmitter of thought provided by a cognitive process of condensation through which complex conceptual structures are distilled to their core. *Condensation* is the process by which multiple pieces of information are compressed into a single, coherent idea or image within the mind, inviting the subjects to venture on an intellectual and emotional journey that transcends time and space and echoes the very nature of human cognition.

This book embarks on the exploration of the interconnection between our cognitive endeavors and the iconic power that gives strength to the short story—a power that resides in its ability to evoke profound cultural, emotional, and intellectual connections. The term *iconic power* refers to the compelling and enduring impact that short stories hold over our collective imagination and cultural consciousness. Short stories possess the ability to distill complex themes, perceptions, emotions, and cultural nuances into concise narratives, connecting deeply with readers and leaving an indelible mark on their thoughts and feelings. As we study the realm of the short story, we reveal a world where the literary mind finds its reflection, and where the art of storytelling becomes a mirror of the different cognitive processes that shape our understanding of the world and our place within it. This exploration deepens into the intersections of culture, cognition, and affective resonance, shedding light on the interwoven threads Story, Metaphoric Understanding and Schemas that bind literature to the complex world of thought and experience.

The linguistic and literary study of cognitive issues follows a methodology that depends, in part, on whether we want to characterize how individuals use cognitive devices in context (corpus linguistics, discourse analysis) or whether we are interested in making hypotheses concerning our shared conceptual system (the lexical approach). The former can be regarded as a "bottom-up" approach, while the latter as a "top-down" one (Kövecses, 2019). In this research, we use both approaches, the lexical approach, and the corpus-based approach, using a corpus arranged randomly (see Annex). The lexical might fall short in an approximation to the iconic power of what is studied here. We search for various lexical items or other types of information that are related to specific subject matters. The sources for the lexical approach are monolingual and bilingual dictionaries, thesauri, collocation dictionaries, idiom dictionaries of various sorts, and, in general, any collections of words and phrases related to a concept. The various lexical items that belong to a particular concept, or, as it is commonly referred to in cognitive linguistics, a domain, are *types*, not tokens. The types provided by the dictionaries represent the most conventionalized linguistic items of a language related to a domain, but they are *decontextualized*. Opposite to them are the *contextualized linguistic expressions*, that is, *tokens*, given by the expressions in their context (Kövecses, 2019). One of the limitations here would be an explicit separation between types and tokens in the argumentations presented. The reader may consider solving them bearing this in mind.

This book is, thus, a comprehensive cognitive linguistic exploration of Seamus Heaney which unfolds across a thoughtfully structured series of chapters reflecting the interplay of culture, cognition, and affective engagement within his captivating works. Its chapters provide a refined analysis of the short story and of Heaney's profound themes and narrative techniques, shedding light on the multifaceted dimensions of his literary creations.

The chapters unfold as follows:

> Chapter 1: Introduction.
>
> Chapter 2: The Subject. In this foundational chapter, the book proceeds by examining the concept of "The Subject in Poetry" through a cognitive lens. It introduces the reader to a cognitive approach and uses cognitive poetics as tools for analyzing Heaney's work. It provides the concept of a poem as a short story, blurring the traditional boundaries between poetry and prose narrative. While poetry and short stories are distinct literary forms, they share common elements in their exploration of themes, characters, emotions, and human experiences, and both forms share a common goal: to engage readers, evoke emotions, and offer insights into the human condition. Viewing a poem as a short story allows for a deeper appreciation of its iconic and storytelling aspects.
>
> Chapter 3: The Iconic Power of the Short Story. This chapter serves as a cornerstone, showing the essence of the short story form and its profound impact. It dissects the structure of short stories and presents the notion of the short story as fundamental for the human mind. Furthermore, it explores how culture interplays with the iconicity inherent in the short story, elucidating the crossroads of narrative and cultural significance.
>
> Chapter 4: Metaphor and the Cognitive Phenomenon. This chapter unfolds the fascinating realm of metaphor and its cognitive implications. It scrutinizes the cognitive and affective involvement

that metaphors elicit, seeing the synesthetic metaphors that Heaney artfully weaves into his narratives.

Chapter 5: Textual Analysis. The heart of the book lies in this chapter, where it conducts detailed textual analysis of select works by Seamus Heaney. The sub-chapters meticulously dissect and interpret specific stories under the format of poems, namely "The First Words," "Remembered Columns," "Lint Water" and "Sruth." Through these analyzes, the book uncovers the layers of meaning, cultural resonances, and cognitive underpinnings embedded within each narrative.

Chapter 6: Final Remarks and Conclusions. The book culminates in its concluding chapter where readers are offered a synthesis of findings and insights. It encapsulates the overarching significance of culture, cognition, and affective involvement within Heaney's work, underlining the enduring impact of his literary contributions.

All in all, "The Iconic Power of Short Story: Exploring Culture, Cognition, and Affective Involvement in Seamus Heaney" traverses the terrain of literature, cognition, and culture, unraveling Seamus Heaney's narrative prowess. Altogether, this book provides a compelling and illuminating journey for those seeking a deeper understanding of the interplay between human experience and literary expression.

CHAPTER 2

The Subject

2.1 The Subject in Poetry

> Poetry should be great and unobtrusive, a thing which enters into one's soul, and does not startle or amaze with itself, but with its subject. (John Keats. Letter to John Hamilton Reynolds, February 3, 1818)

Following Keats (see Rollins, 2012: 80–85) in his memorable words, and knowing the considerable influence he had on Seamus Heaney, the main question we must ask ourselves would be "what is the subject?" Does the poetic text need to have a subject? If the words are not easily understood and the theme, the object of the poem, is not easily understood either, or is not given to the reader, what does he or she get out of it, how does he or she resolve it, and why is it presented to him or her the way it is?

According to Hughes (1993: 47), in *The Haw Lantern* (Heaney, 1987), for example, there is a movement from everyday experience to allegory that informs us as a parable, a story told as an example to teach or explain something. In that everyday experience silence and inarticulateness form the center of the action. But each poem, like any allegory or parable, possesses a concrete subject in itself.

"Saying and representing things" (Fennell, 1991: 9), is the main part of the discourse. But today there is a general tendency towards reticence, an adjective that describes a phenomenon that catches our attention and that I have found very interesting indeed. I refer to reticence in the sense of saying something half-heartedly or implying that one is keeping quiet about something one should or could say. That is, of reserve. This word describes an attitude reflected in a great number of poets and to some extent characteristic of the poet that is the center of this study. Saying little and with reluctance would be what traditionally characterizes the discourse of any poet who does not have a concrete subject in his or her poetry or who wants to keep it out of sight.

Two kinds of reticent text can be found. That which deploys many possibilities of interpretation, in order not to commit itself to a particular theme, or that in which a theme is set forth as so commonplace and general that it conveys nothing beyond mere words. The latter we can illustrate with the following example given by Crystal (1988: 133):

> Almost anything
> Can be made to look
> Poetic,
> As long as it is
> Written in lines.

As Crystal (1988: 136) suggests, poetic diction, style, the breaking of rules, are at the service of the poet to imprint identity on the writing, and to show an inner vision from a certain perspective. And this process is not done at random, nor arbitrarily. At each point, with each example, there is a theme that gives unity, that unifies and converts the poem into a communicative whole.

Heaney himself speaks of the reticence characteristic of Northern Irish public discourse (Heaney, 1988) and the reason why this feature of his poetry is so striking to us is that it is not mere reticence but a kind of silence that operates according to rules predetermined perhaps by that particular framework and unknown to us for the time being (Fennell, 1991).

The recurrent use of the theme of silence and inarticulateness or inability to express, as well as Heaney's view of speech as a dangerous activity, define his work within the first of the established categories regarding the reticent poetic text (Fennell, 1991). Heaney loved language, loved the use of every word, sought the beauty of language, but feared the meaning that may be hidden beneath it when it is made public. Thus, sharing his people's conception of public speech as dangerous since, traditionally, the minority of Northern Ireland's Catholics were characterized by caution, care in what they said and how they behaved, in vigilance.

Seamus Heaney, born in County Derry into a family belonging to the Catholic minority in Northern Ireland, never chose the path of belligerence, although his land is always immersed in problems of that nature. His poetic skill, precision and energy characterize the poetic language of his first stage, in which nature is always present, but turn into a public voice more bitter, more ironic and, above all, less confident latter on. Heaney's first verses, somewhat overloaded and sober, developed thanks to his avid reading and assimilation of the Movement poets of the 1950s (e.g., Gunn's macho tone or Ted Hughes's taste for nature in its most violent and cruel aspects), the slow technique and the calm and intimate tone of the American Roethke, as well as the incorporation of a kind of free indirect style adopted from poetry or from some turns and words of regional speech, which perfected his technique and style (Hughes, 1993). In his work Heaney uses the familiar, the everyday, as a pretext to advance towards the apprehension of the intuited and the mysterious. But while any such inquiry gives us the sense of being a journey inward and inward (Longley, 1994), as we shall see in the metaphors that will be discussed later on, he pictures a miraculous outside world as a result.

Heaney, a great lover and connoisseur of language, and often user of unusual words or expressions and archaisms, was a master of austerity, which keeps the reader at a certain distance, probably intentionally (Parker, 1993). His tone was serious, and at times can even be considered somewhat lugubrious. Very rarely did he include a touch of extra light or color, and certainly never humor. His work lacks everything that would supposedly make it easy to win over the audience, although he definitely succeeded without needing to resort to such.

Heaney often gave the impression that he restrained himself, that he chose with great care not only the words he used but also what he wished to reveal about himself. After all, it was he who from his "Land of the Unspoken" gave the curious antiphon or motet "whatever you say, say nothing." The poem reminds the reader of the paradox of a writer who, throughout his life, extols language, but at the same time acts with great caution because he knows the harm that language can do. Or more specifically, the damage that language as discourse, and especially when public, can do.

When everyday life is applied to poetic discourse, the meaning of it will come to be modified by different contexts (Higgins, 2021), but at the same time its effect endures in everyday life to enable, disable, or prescribe certain modes of speech and certain subjects. When the belief of the

Catholics of County Derry, where Heaney came from, that public speech is potentially harmful is applied to poetry to be published in London or New York, public speech varies its meaning from speech for individuals outside the domestic sphere to speech for educated speakers of English in general. And for both the poet and the farmer, his maxim provides them with a practical guide to finding a way to keep themselves safe, as well as forms of public discourse that, while avoiding harm to self or others, will benefit all.

Between the reality described and our expectations there is a cognitive void, an incongruence. The human condition, everyday events, the state of the country or the world, men, women, history, the future, nature, beauty, fear, love, death, and so many other general themes are eluded and instead the poet speaks of particular themes, of himself, of his feelings and memories, of incidents that occurred in his domestic and family life. Heaney's desired effect is to avoid saying anything "concrete" and for that he talks about the life, thoughts, or intentions of the individual, about family, community. Searching for trivial and unimportant topics and the absence of concrete assertions, using evasive resources, without peripheral, convoluted contents, ambiguity, half words, incongruous anecdotes, etc., provide the *subject without subject* and characterize the speaking self, amid the turbulent social and political landscapes of Ireland (Curtis, 1985; Vendler, 1998; O'Brien, 2002).

By avoiding making pronouncements on general topics, he avoids saying things that might lead people to believe or act wrongly, he avoids entering any kind of controversy (Vendler, 1998), but perhaps by avoiding doing harm he does a very modest good. Precisely because his poetry is silent, not by accident but by the poet's own desire, it contains an inner tension that fascinates his readers, a compressed intensity, an opaque clarity that envelops the reader. And after a moment's reflection he confirms that neither rural life, nor everyday life, nor the conflict in Northern Ireland, are really the subjects of his poems, but rather scenes or incidents remembered by the poet—accompanied by his feelings—, which is not accepted by the interpreter, who sees through those particular issues so that they represent something more than their particular content. Poetry can do this with feelings, with pictorial scenes and sensorial incidents, it can, through condensation, create meaning and resonate in our minds.

The success of his poetry lies not only in what he says or represents expressly (Andrews, 1992; Vendler, 1995), but in what he suggests, intentionally or for any other reason—external to the poet, related to the reader, or to the world around us. The reader perceives an image, notices presences, absences and emphases, internalizes values and evaluations. The most striking elements of the image of the world that Heaney presents in his poetry are materialism and non-transcendentality; a world that is mainly rural and silent, without people in its landscapes; the goodness of the material earth, the primordial mud, and the rustic past, of work, of marriage, of friendship, and of family rootedness; the sadness and evil of violent death; the compulsive pulse of an individual's cultural roots and tribal reminiscences; the dubious value of commitment outside the domestic sphere; and the highly suspect or dangerous power of communal or patriotic loyalty. The one major public issue that stands out for any interpreter, the conflict in Northern Ireland, is portrayed, impressionistically, as a dreary realm in which the vigilantes, soldiers, police and prisons of the rational state flourish.

The I or self from which the poems unfold shows an introspective view of an educated country man, who wore rubber boots and sloshed through the mud of his ever-wet countryside. A man who delighted in words, in earthly things, who was tender, committed and occasionally angry about public issues, but who stayed,—perhaps feeling deep down guilty—, out of action; who supported Amnesty International; who paid attention to his traditions and his roots; who refrained humbly and shrewdly from making pronouncements on human life or on issues to do with people or with the homeland and its conflicts. The "I" of the poem in Heaney stands for the "I" of the poet who is writing (O'Brien, 2002: 153).

At times, his poems contain difficult words and Irish allusions or expressions, and his verses have no special musical melody. But it is precisely this humble or almost austere silence of the poet that most pleases the academics. Meaning little or nothing has effectively become the defining characteristic of contemporary poetry, of Heaney's poetry and of the doctrine that this is how poetry should be in a justification of reality (see Corcoran, 1986, 2008, 2014; Corcoran and Heaney, 1998; O'Donoghue, 2017; Vendler, 1992, 1998; Kiberd, 2005: 232; O'Brien, 2002: 154). When a poem is said to be about poetry the word poetry is often used to mean many things: how people construct something intelligible out of random experiences; how people choose to express what they love and so many other things. Though that sensibility and temperament have been influenced by the historical possibilities of the author's context, what a poem ultimately symbolizes is not the outer world but rather the sensibility and temperament shaped by that context (Longley, 1994).

Heaney therefore captures a certain historical period by reflecting a sensibility. The poem encompasses the outside world, which serves as the inspiration for its imagery, metaphors, symbols, myths, and, of course, its linguistic structure and lexical choices, but it does so in order to color mentally it all and erase the world, its surrounds, and all of creation from inside its own psyche, because as Andrew Marvell puts it in his poem "The Garden" and Heaney points out in his book *The Government of the Tongue* (1988), "The mind, that ocean where each kind/Doth straight its own resemblance find;/Yet it creates, transcending these,/Far other worlds and other seas,/Annihilating all that's made/To a green thought in a green shade" (lines 41–48).

Other scholars have equated a poem to the mind (Gibbs, 1994; Turner, 1991, 1996). A poem is similar to, and represents, the mind function in its medium, like a witty speech or an externalized understanding. But this is not to say that the poet's mind matches what the interpreter's mind receives. This cognitive view of the poetic product does not support poetry of ideas, meaning something concrete, saying something, to be communicated directly to the interpreter. But neither can we support a conception of the ideal poem described as an unfinished thought in active language or a vigorous verbal reflection. Additionally, because language serves as the conduit for poetry and since language cannot fail to communicate when utilized in accordance with any of the conceivable encoding rules, and even inconceivable ones, there doesn't seem to be any need to be concerned about the transmission of poetry itself. As time passes, all poetry gets easier. Thus, there is no need to stress about speaking for everyone or being universal (Heaney, 1988).

It is a question of how we conceptualize poetry and how it is described, which, although published to large audiences can have said nothing about general issues, and then it would cancel itself out as genuine public discourse.

It would be a reflection addressed to the I or self and, as such, poetry at its best. In Heaney, the poet's "I" is somehow detached from ordinary social circumstances, reserved for solipsistic meditations, thoughtfully entranced or as if in a Calderonian dream. In an occidental civilization that boasts of its social awareness and democratic culture, Heaney was aware that his conviction that public discourse is dangerous and perhaps detrimental kept him from performing good deeds for others, as such expected deeds may be accomplished through the public discourse of his poems.

Heaney stated the following in the last paragraph of his inaugural lecture as Professor of Poetry at Oxford University in 1989 entitled "The Redress of Poetry" (see Fennell, 1991: 42):

> [Poetry] has to withstand as well as to envisage, and in order to do so it must contain within itself the coordinates of the reality which surrounds it and out of which it is engendered. When it does contain these coordinates, it becomes a power to which we can have redress: it functions as the rim of the silence out of which consciousness arrives and into which it must descend. For a moment, we can remember ourselves as fully empowered beings.

The metaphor at work in saying "the rim of the silence out of which consciousness arrives and into which it must descend" revolves around a figure and a ground, the concept of poetry as a "rim" and "silence" as the context. The "rim" implies a boundary or threshold, while "silence" represents a state of absence of sound or external noise. This metaphor suggests that poetry marks the edge or boundary of silence, separating the inner world of consciousness from the external realm of noise. The combination of "rim" and "silence" can evoke sensory associations that show the usual synesthetic power of his writings. Readers might imagine the quietness of silence and the sense of transition as we approach a "rim," creating a subtle synesthetic experience of stillness and boundary. The phrase blends the metaphorical concept of poetry as a "rim" with the context of "silence." The blending creates a cognitive whole that emphasizes the role of poetry in relation to consciousness. Just as a rim defines the edge of something, poetry defines the boundary between silence and consciousness. It tells a story that locates us in progression, that is, in movement, in a journey. The phrase carries emotional resonance by invoking the idea of consciousness emerging from silence and descending back into it. This journey from silence to consciousness and back again touches on themes of introspection, thought, and reflection. It might evoke a sense of contemplation or even a certain depth of emotion as readers reflect on the concept of consciousness and silence.

Consciousness might be considered the opposite of silence if we recall our interior voice echoing. Not all conscious experiences are articulated as an ongoing inner voice, they can include images, sensations, feelings. But if we think about a non-silent conscious situation, we can immediately evoke our inner voice. An interior voice or interior monologue in a story is often referred to as "stream of consciousness." Stream of consciousness is a narrative technique that presents a character's thoughts, feelings, and perceptions as they occur in their mind, often in an unfiltered and continuous manner. This technique aims to mimic the flow of a character's inner thoughts, providing insight into their inner workings and creating a more immersive reading experience.

Following this notion, we can say that Heaney envisions poetry as a journey to consciousness (conceptual metaphor POETRY IS A JOURNEY) with a departure point, a path and a destination. A journey for our consciousness, that is what makes us become in our minds empowered beings (Heaney, 1988).

With this description we can envision how the short story shapes our journeys. It provides beginning, middle and end (basic cognitive structure SOURCE, PATH, GOAL) providing conscious and sometimes unconscious experiences. Within its journey, the story provides presentation, knot (or body) and resolution, giving our mind the power to understand and to be. In essence, this draws parallels between Heaney's conceptualization of the poetic journey and the transformative nature of storytelling, with a beginning, a middle and an end. Both poetry and storytelling guide readers on cognitive and emotional journeys, empowering them to explore new realms of understanding and contributing to their growth as perceptive and reflective beings.

The metaphors POETRY IS A JOURNEY and STORYTELLING IS A JOURNEY can indeed be traced back to a primary, foundational metaphor that underlies both. This foundational metaphor, derived from our primary embodied experiences, is the more general concept of life as a journey (LIFE IS A JOURNEY) (Lakoff and Johnson, 1980, 1999). Both poetry and storytelling draw upon this fundamental metaphor to create their specific variations. The metaphor of life as a journey is deeply ingrained in human thought and language. It is a concept that resonates across cultures and languages, reflecting our understanding of the progression, experiences, and challenges we encounter throughout our lives. Both variations of this primary metaphor build upon the core idea of progression, experiences, and meaningful transitions, whether within the context of reading a poem or engaging with a short narrative. This shared cognitive foundation highlights the power of the short story shaping our understanding of complex ideas and facilitating our engagement with various forms of artistic expression.

Heaney envisions poetry as a transformative journey that engages the reader's consciousness and empowers the mind (see Fennell, 1991: 42). A similar framework can be applied to the structure and impact of a story:

1. Departure Point and Presentation: In Heaney's vision of poetry, the departure point signifies the beginning of a transformative journey. Similarly, in storytelling, the presentation of characters, setting, and initial circumstances provides the departure point for the reader's journey into the narrative world. This introduction sets the stage for the reader to embark on a mental exploration.
2. Path and Knot: The path in Heaney's metaphorical journey involves the exploration of different layers of meaning and connections within the poem. Similarly, in a story, the development of plot, conflicts, and interactions between characters creates the path that the reader follows. The knot (or body) represents the complexities and challenges encountered along the way, echoing the conflicts that characters face in a story's narrative.
3. Destination and Resolution: Just as Heaney's journey leads to a destination where new understandings are achieved, a story culminates in the resolution. This is the point where the narrative threads are woven together, conflicts are addressed, and the reader gains insights into the characters and their journey. This

resolution, like the destination in Heaney's metaphor, allows the reader to synthesize the journey's meaning.

Heaney suggests that the metaphorical journey through poetry empowers the reader's mind by engaging with layers of meaning and opening up new perspectives. A well-crafted story has the potential to engage the reader's mind, enabling them to empathize with characters, explore themes, and gain insights that can influence their own perspectives. The aim of the journey, call it indistinctly poem or story, is thus the empowerment of the mind.

Heaney followed Frost and Eliot, saying that poetry houses older and deeper levels of energy than those supplied by explicit meaning and immediate rhythmic stimulus (Heaney, 1988: 148), and also Lowell, saying that poems are events rather than the records of events (Heaney, 1988: 151):

> Read it a hundred times but it will never lose its impression of a meaning once unfolded by surprise. It begins in delight, bends to impulse, assumes its direction with the first line discovered, runs along a path of fortunate events, and ends in a clarification of life.

Heaney talks about "redress" in his works. He follows the OED in the first sense that it provides for the noun: "Reparation of, satisfaction or compensation for, a wrong sustained or the loss resulting from this" and for the verb as "To set (a person or thing) upright again; to raise again to an erected position. Also fig. to set up again, restore, re-establish." However, he states that poetry goes beyond redress because its force is not just cultural or political, but also surprising and reliable as it enters our field of vision and animates our physical and intelligent being becoming a matter of finding "a course for the breakaway of innate capacity, a course where something unhindered, yet directed, can sweep ahead into its full potential" (Heaney, 1995: 15).

Even in his early more overtly political poems, he seeks neutrality, because he does not want his work to become a mere denunciation or a propaganda weapon, but neither does he turn his back on reality. His desire to iron out differences is characteristic, and he has never entirely lost his faith in the ability of art to soothe, to bring relief and comfort, but it is very difficult to deal with literature, and especially Irish literature, without being drawn into issues of culture and politics (Longley, 1994). So, true to the trajectory of all his writing, Heaney uses the familiar, the everyday, as a pretext—almost in a literal sense "pre-text" to move towards apprehension of the intuited and the mysterious (Hughes, 1993: 50).

We can see it all in his poem "From the Frontier of Writing" (lines 13–18):

> So you drive on to the frontier of writing
> where it happens again. The guns on tripods;
> the sergeant with his on-off mike repeating
>
> data about you, waiting for the squawk
> of clearance; the marksman training down
> out of the sun upon you like a hawk.

The dreamed world is not a space of absolute and unconditional freedom, a kind of paradise of individualism still called "liberal" (that is, of bourgeois "laissez faire") but an ideal space of conscience where the writer freely assumes the onerous responsibility of putting his gift at the service of the community. It is symptomatic of this attitude that Heaney, who, as we have seen, never allowed his work to become a pure denunciation or a propaganda weapon, but neither did he turn his back on the reality of the Irish carnage, but chose this moment to donate one of his poems to Amnesty International. The poem "From the Republic of Conscience" published by Amnesty International on World Human Rights Day in 1985 (included in his book *The Haw Lantern*) finds with the other political and ethical allegories the most convenient context. Simplicity is not simplicity; the poem, with its unfussy dignity and homespun wisdom, recalls the best Hardy and a little of Antonio Machado (Hughes, 1993). Heaney throughout his creative life tends to trace the indissoluble links between exterior and interior, that is, between the life of the senses and the mental life. Public life, intimate life, memory, the exemplary value of the poet's conscience, isolation, absence … are intermingled and confused. See his lines in The Republic of Conscience (1–6):

> When I landed in the republic of conscience
> it was so noiseless when the engines stopped
> I could hear a curlew high above the runway.
>
> At immigration, the clerk was an old man
> who produced a wallet from his homespun coat
> and showed me a photograph of my grandfather.

When Heaney refers to a specific place in his poetry, it does not mean that he is referring to a specific geographical space but to an idea (IDEAS ARE LOCATIONS), which he has arrived at through his experience, his previous state, his place of origin, his roots. This way, we could say that what he states in his critical essays (Heaney, 1988: 9) is what he actually intends to show in poems such as "From the Frontier of Writing."

In his famous essay "The Government of the tongue" (1988: 3) he points out the place:

> … it was not so much a matter of attaching oneself to a living symbol of being rooted in the native ground; it was more a matter of preparing to be unrooted, to be spirited away into some transparent, yet indigenous afterlife. The new place was all idea, if you like; it was generated out of my experience of the old place but it was not a topological location. It was and remains an imagined realm, even if it can be located at an earthly spot, a placeless heaven rather than a heavenly place [...]. The horizons of the little fields and hills, whether they are gloomy and constricting or radiant and enhancing, sensed as the horizons of consciousness. Within those horizons, however, the poet who utters the poems is alive and well as a sharp critical intelligence.

According to Heaney (1988), as in the poems of Patrick Kavanagh, the reader realizes that the places described by the poet are places that actually exist in the real landscape and are constantly present in his memory (see Figure 1). The poet's conscious experience of physical reality forces him to create himself, his mind, his poetic identity, and his poems in relation to the horizon around that experience:

> I have learned to value this poetry of inner freedom very highly. It is an example of self-conquest, a style discovered to express this poet's unique response to his universal ordinariness, a way of re-establishing the authenticity of personal experience and surviving as a credible being.

The Subject

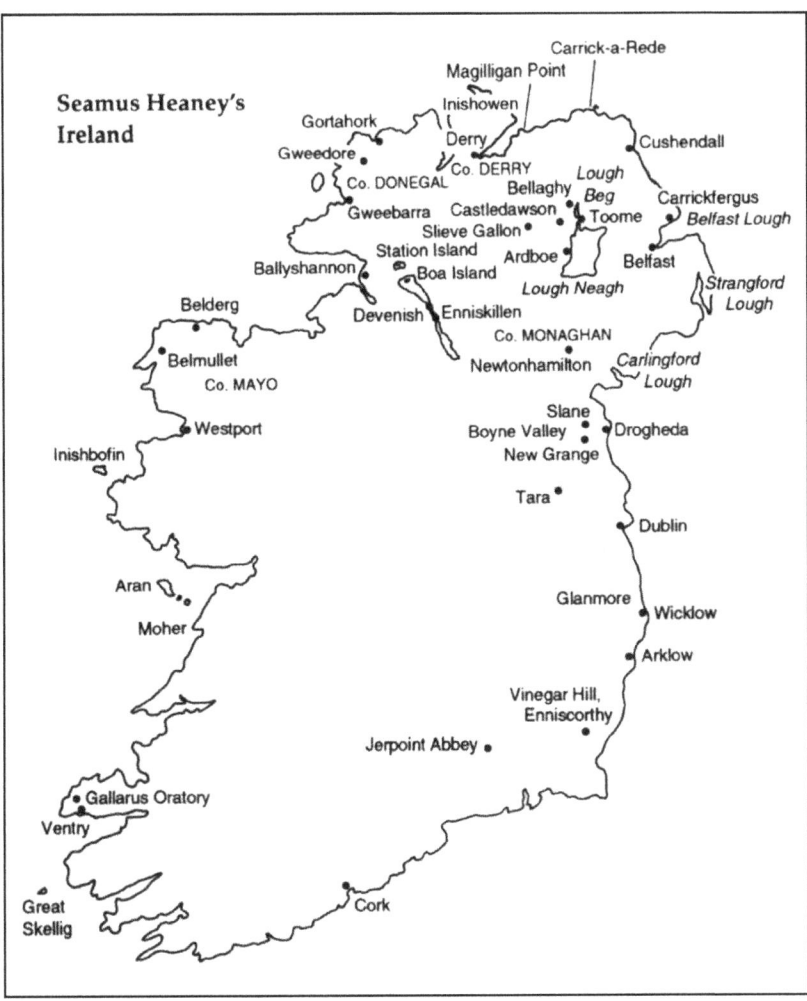

Figure 1. Important geographical locations in Heaney's Ireland (Parker, 1993: xi).

Heaney also speaks of what he means with the phrase "The Government of the Tongue" (1988: 92). It communicates his idea that poetry possesses its own vindicating or justifying force, its own power. A capacity to rule that has been given to the tongue, which stands for the poet's unique ability to communicate as well as the fundamental components of language. Poetic art is seen to have special authority. The self-validating processes we refer to as inspiration cause us, as readers, to bow to the authority of the creative form rather than by force of the ethical and moral exercise of thought. This becomes especially true if we consider inspiration to be a psychosomatic phenomenon in which the poet transforms into a receiver of the voices of the world and a vehicle for expressing both his own subconscious and the collective subconscious for a moment before losing those possessions once the moment has passed.

Poetry has the ability to facilitate new and mediated ways of connection between our nature and the nature of the world we live in Heaney (1988: 93). The earliest proof of this attitude appeared in the Greek conception that when a poet raised his or her voice, it was the voice of a god speaking, and the twentieth century has been characterized by this frame of mind. Any interference with a totally unbiased cognitions of the form-seeking imagination by intellectual knowledge is poetic sabotage, an insult to the governing and executing powers of expression itself. Being part of the creative process and the states in which it takes place provides poetry with an enormous power, that would never disappear because even if you read it a hundred times, the poem will never lose its impression of a meaning once unfolded by surprise. Influenced by Frost, Heaney says the following about poetry (Heaney, 1988: 93):

> It begins in delight, it inclines to the impulse, it assumes direction with the first line laid down, it runs a course of lucky events and ends in a clarification of life— not necessarily a great clarification, such as sects and cults are founded on, but in a momentary stay against confusion.

And he goes further arguing that (Heaney, 1988: 94) "Art is not an inferior reflection of some ordained heavenly system but a rehearsal of it in earthly terms; art does not trace the given map of a better reality but improvises an inspired sketch of it."

As a whole, Heaney provides a definition of poetry allowing focus in that place (LOCATION) between what will happen and what we want to happen; it serves not as a diversion but as pure concentration (FORCE), a focus where our strength of concentration causes us to concentrate on ourselves. This location resembles an abyss that implies endless possibilities and that sometimes is not crossed, because it is more comfortable for us to stay on the side of a random possibility or even to stay on the side of what we would like it to mean, and then we adapt and play with the meaning in order to bring it to our terrain or primitive/personal idea. It is an attitude typical of human beings that once an approach or an idea is chosen or considered as true, they look for all possible reasonings and arguments in favor of it and try to refute, deny, ignore or even omit any that does not fit them or that does not fit their initial approach. Words have power (FORCE) to lead us through possible journeys (STORIES), but governing words (their force) allows them to become a portal (CONTAINER):

> This gives poetry its governing power [...]. Poetry is more a threshold than a path, one constantly approached and constantly departed from, at which reader and writer undergo in their different ways the experience of being at the same time summoned and released. (Heaney, 1988: 108)

The force within words possesses the ability to guide us on potential narratives, yet when wielded with control, these words are transformed into a conduit. This attribute bestows poetry with its authority. Rather than a linear route, poetry embodies a threshold continuously approached and left behind, where both reader and writer undergo the unique encounter of being simultaneously beckoned and set free, as insightfully expressed by Heaney (1988: 108). The subject revolves then around the concept of the influential power held by words and around how words can guide us through journeys and stories, and when managed effectively, they achieve such transformation.

2.2 The Cognitive Linguistic Approach

2.2.1 Definition and Scope

The Cognitive Linguistic Approach (CLA) is a comprehensive framework that plays a fundamental role in understanding both human language and thought. The approach elaborated for the purpose of this book was designed to enhance our comprehension of various aspects of cognition and linguistic expression. It offers a structured and cohesive set of principles, strategies, and methods that can be effectively applied in different fields, ranging from linguistics to education and beyond. This CLA serves as a theoretical foundation for tasks like textual analysis and literary criticism, providing insights into how language is intimately connected with human cognition and perception. Beyond its theoretical value, this CLA also offers practical benefits. It can be applied in different fields and employed to formulate instructional activities, plan lessons, and foster student engagement, making it particularly valuable in the realm of education and pedagogy.

In the context of this book, which focuses on the analysis of Seamus Heaney's work, the CLA is both defined and systematically applied. This initial chapter establishes a clear definition of the CLA frame and its relevance to the analysis of literature. It shows various cognitive aspects in depth, systematically examining how Heaney's writings embody and reflect cognitive principles. The methodological application, put into practice in Chapter 4, encompasses the overarching philosophy and guiding principles that underlie human cognition. Using the CLA in this book not only helps us explore Heaney's literary works but also provides a broader perspective on how language and thought are interconnected. In doing so, it sheds light on the fundamental mechanisms that shape the human mind and cognition, contributing to a richer understanding of both literature and cognitive processes.

The Cognitive Linguistic Approach departs from traditional cognitive linguistics (Lakoff and Johnson, 1980; Lakoff and Turner, 1989) and cognitive poetics (Freeman, 2010; Bretones et al., 2021) by providing a more specialized and structured approach tailored for textual analysis and literary exploration. Cognitive linguistics is the branch of linguistics that examines human cognition within a theory of mind, aiming to elucidate the overarching principles that govern all facets of human thought and provide a comprehensive framework that encompasses language, mind, and brain. Moving beyond Cartesian dualism and the division of mind and body, cognitivism offers an alternative vantage point to analyze the intricate phenomenon of human language (Lakoff and Johnson, 1999). It considers language as a human general instrument that helps us understand the world (Bretones, 2001, 2005; Barsalou, 1999, 2008; Gallese and Lakoff, 2005; Tomasello, 2008).

In this context, embodiment is a key concept because it refers to the idea that human cognition is fundamentally shaped by the sensory-motor experiences of the body interacting with the environment. This perspective contrasts with traditional views that consider cognition as an abstract, symbolic manipulation of mental representations. Embodiment posits that our understanding of concepts, language, and even abstract reasoning is grounded in our bodily experiences and interactions with the physical world (Lakoff and Johnson, 1999). For instance, since our brain cannot file all the perceptual information it receives, we use strategies such as the segregation of the information between figure and background. This cognitive process has been labeled as *profiling* by Langacker (1987), or *windows of attention* by Talmy (2000) and makes understanding possible. Another important assumption in cognitive linguistics is that specific sensorial experiences, such as color, are experienced differently by speakers of different languages (Boroditsky, 2000, 2011). For example, take the case of speakers of Russian and Spanish, who have separate words for light and dark blue, being quicker at discriminating between light and dark blue compared to English speakers. Each language requires a certain mental structure in connection to the language, an arrangement that can shape how we mentally represent and interpret visual information and concepts. So, language and culture shape the way we perceive and understand the world (Bretones et al., 2021: 10).

Cognitive linguistics provides specific tools, *cognitive tools*, that is, mental processes, strategies, or mechanisms used by humans in systematic and recurrent ways to facilitate various cognitive tasks such as learning, problem-solving, reasoning, memory retrieval, and communication. These tools help individuals interact with information, make sense of their environment, and navigate complex cognitive challenges. Cognitive tools can be both external, such as physical objects or technologies,—which with the intention of avoiding confusion will be called here cognitive artifacts—, and internal, referring to mental processes and strategies. Cognitive tools play a crucial role in shaping how humans process information and engage with the world around them.

2.2.2 Cognitive Tools

Cognitive tools are instruments used by humans to construct meaning, understand language, and engage in cognitive activities. Cognitive linguistics emphasizes the role of these tools in shaping how we perceive and conceptualize the world, as well as in how we use language to express our thoughts and experiences. Some cognitive tools, as understood within the framework of Cognitive Linguistics, are:

1. Metaphor: Metaphor is a cognitive tool that allows us to understand one concept in terms of another by mapping the structure of one domain (source or input 1) onto another domain (target or input 2) (Lakoff and Johnson, 1980). For example, understanding "We're approaching the deadline" involves the use of the TIME IS PATH metaphor, which helps us understand linear movement towards a time destination.
2. Image Schema: Image schemas are recurring spatial and motor patterns that serve as fundamental building blocks of meaning (Lakoff and Johnson, 1999). For example, CONTAINER OR PATH are image schemas that contribute to our understanding of various abstract concepts, for example, of love in "I am in love."
3. Blending: Conceptual blending involves merging elements from different mental spaces to create new meaning (Fauconnier and Turner, 2002). It is a cognitive tool that enables us to create novel and often metaphorical concepts and that provides conceptual integration (see Figure 2). For example, understanding "He's digging his own grave" involves the conceptual integration of a prototypical digger and a gravedigger, none of them providing or implying any harmful effect until the blend incorporates emergent meaning turning the action into a potentially damaging one for the subject.
4. Prototype: Prototype theory posits that categories are organized around prototypes or typical exemplars (Rosch, 1978). This cognitive tool helps us understand and categorize concepts based on their typical features and central examples. The central meaning

The Subject

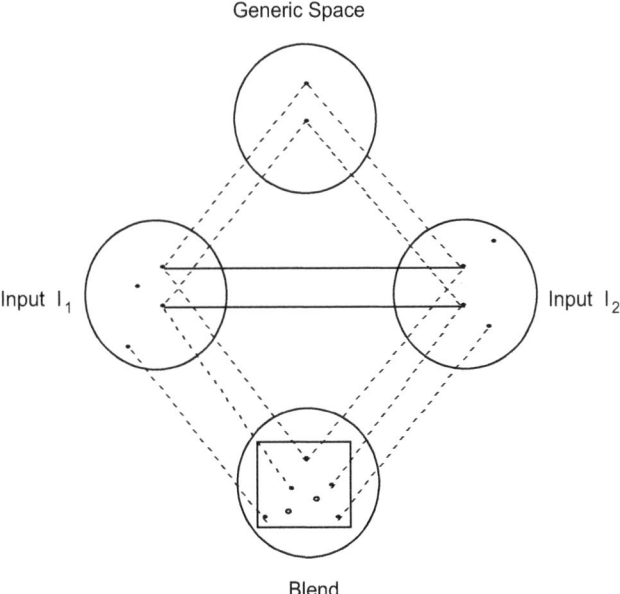

Figure 2. Basic diagram representing the process of blending (Fauconnier and Turner, 2002: 46).

    for a digger would be a prototypical "person who excavates or turns up the earth with a mattock, spade, or other tool" (OED).

5. Radial Network: Radial categories are structured around a central prototype and extend outward to include less central members (Rosch, 1978; Lakoff, 1987). This cognitive tool allows for flexible and dynamic categorization. For instance, we easily access the central meaning of digger through its prototypical sense (normally accessible as the first sense given to it in dictionaries,— see above OED), but in connection to this sense other meanings can come to mind such as diggeress ("a female digger; a digger's wife," OED), gravedigger ("one whose employment it is to dig graves," OED), gold-digger ("a person who digs for gold" OED) or gold-digger ("figurative. colloquial (originally US) a person (originally and esp. a woman) who forms for profit a romantic or sexual relationship with another person …," OED).

6. Frame: Frames are cognitive structures that represent our knowledge about a particular concept or situation. Frame semantics helps us understand how different aspects of meaning are activated in different contexts (Fillmore, 1982). They provide the information that enables meaning salience within semantic networks. For example, if we face the expression "digging up," the frame allows discrimination of a regular transitive action meaning "To take or get out of the ground, etc., by digging or excavating" or "to exhume, disinter, unearth" (OED) or "figurative to obtain, find, search …" (OED).
7. Force Dynamics: It is a cognitive tool used to conceptualize and express relationships of force, effort, and motion in a metaphorical way. It plays a role in how we understand and express causation, agency, and control inside the frame (Talmy, 2000, 2003). For instance, the "up" in the expression "digging up" would describe a force and motion metaphorically understood, different to that of the conventional action of a person digging, normally pushing mainly downwards.
8. Embodied Simulation: Embodied cognition considers how our bodily experiences and sensorimotor interactions with the world shape our conceptual understanding and language use (Lakoff, 2012). We achieve this understanding through mental simulation (Barsalou, 1999, 2020). When you think about the action of digging, your brain can activate a network of sensory and motor regions that are associated with the physical act of digging. This is because of the brain's capacity to simulate actions and experiences in response to certain cues, even when you are not actually performing the action: Thinking about the action of digging can trigger the activation of the (i) motor cortex, brain region responsible for planning, coordinating, and executing voluntary movements. When you think about digging, your motor cortex might simulate the neural pathways that would be engaged if you were actually holding a shovel and moving it through the soil. Your (ii) brain's sensory regions may also be engaged. You might mentally recreate the tactile sensations associated with

digging, such as the feeling of the shovel's handle in your hands, the resistance of the soil as you push the shovel into the ground or the texture of the earth against your skin. Your brain might also generate (iii) visual images related to digging. You might mentally see the hole forming in the ground, the movement of the soil, and the shovel's trajectory in "digging." This involves the brain's visual processing regions. When thinking about digging, your brain might activate (iv) proprioception, that is, your sense of the relative position of different parts of your body, allowing you mentally to experience the positions and movements of your limbs as if you were digging. Your brain might also consider the (v) environmental context of digging, such as the location, weather, and surroundings combined with (vi) encyclopedic information stored in your memory (cultural issues). This can involve sensory aspects like the smell of the freshly worked soil or the sounds of the surroundings while digging combined with (vii) emotional associations, such as memories of past experiences involving digging or thoughts about why you might be digging. These associations can further enhance the richness of your sensory-motor activation and are the way in which the brain creates a mental simulation of the action, based on your previous experiences and knowledge. This process allows you to mentally explore and understand actions without physically performing them in that moment.

9. Synesthetic Force: This cognitive tool provides the ability of introducing sensorial experiences (when one sensory or cognitive pathway triggers an involuntary experience in another or enriched sensorial experience) to influence a person's perception, cognition, or creativity. This influence might involve the blending, which can lead to novel ways of perceiving or thinking about the world.

These cognitive tools, as conceived by cognitive linguistics, illustrate how interconnected our mental processes and linguistic expressions are. They offer insights into how humans construct meaning, create language, and make sense of the world around them based on their cognitive capacities and experiences.

2.2.3 Synesthesia as a Cognitive Tool

Synesthesia can be thought of as a unique cognitive phenomenon that blurs the traditional boundaries between sensory and cognitive pathways. It involves the coactivation or intermixing of sensorial experiences, which can lead to a noticeably richer and more interconnected perception and understanding of the world. While synesthesia itself is not considered a deliberate cognitive device in the way that, for example, memory or attention are, it can be considered a distinctive cognitive tool which provides sensorial information coming from different levels to be processed and integrated by the brain.

Synesthetic Force provides the capacity of synesthetic experiences or synesthetic elements to influence or enhance certain cognitive or creative processes. In the context of synesthesia and cognitive linguistics synesthetic force could refer to the ability of synesthetic experiences (where one sensory or cognitive pathway triggers an involuntary experience in another) to influence a person's perception, cognition, or creativity. This influence might involve the blending of sensorial experiences, which can lead to novel ways of perceiving or thinking about the world. For example, in literature or art, synesthetic descriptions can evoke a multisensory experience in the audience, making the work more vivid and impactful. In essence, synesthetic force might be a cognitive tool that provides the capacity of enriching or deepening sensorial human experiences, whether in the realm of perception, cognition, or creativity.

Synesthesia has been considered traditionally as the involuntary physical experience of a cross-modal association, the stimulation of one sensory modality causing a perception in one or more different senses (Cytowic, 1995, 2003, 2024). This type of synesthesia appears to be a left-hemisphere function that is not cortical in the conventional sense, and the hippocampus is critical for its experience. Other approaches to synesthesia considered it a normal brain process that is prematurely displayed to consciousness in a minority of individuals (Bretones, 2001, 2005). Maurice Merleau-Ponty believed that synesthetic perception is the rule and we are unaware of it only because scientific knowledge shifts the center of gravity of experience. Today, different types of synesthesia are widely acknowledged, some considered special neuroatypical conditions that involve various combinations of senses and cognitive processes. Here are a few examples:

- Grapheme-Color Synesthesia: This is one of the most common forms. People with this type of synesthesia perceive letters, numbers, or words as inherently associated with specific colors. For instance, the letter "A" might always appear as red, or the number "4" might be seen always as green.
- Sound-Color Synesthesia: In this type, individuals associate certain sounds or musical notes with specific colors. For example, hearing a specific musical note might trigger the perception of a particular color.
- Spatial Sequence Synesthesia: People with this form of synesthesia perceive numerical sequences as having specific spatial locations. For example, they might see numbers arranged in a mental space where each number has a distinct position.
- Lexical-Gustatory Synesthesia: This form involves experiencing tastes when hearing or reading specific words. Hearing the word "chocolate," for instance, might trigger a taste sensation of chocolate in the synesthete's mouth.
- Mirror-Touch Synesthesia: This type involves feeling physical sensations on one's own body when witnessing another person's tactile experiences. For instance, if someone with mirror-touch synesthesia sees someone being touched on the cheek, they might feel a similar touch on their own cheek.
- Associative Synesthesia: This type involves a more abstract association between stimuli. People might associate certain personality traits with colors, or they might associate specific emotions with certain shapes.

In these cases, synesthesia encompasses distinctive sensory encounters that may not be universally shared and often encompass unforeseen or unconventional links between sensory modalities. This phenomenon stands as an individualistic and distinct occurrence, differing from the broader and collectively comprehended experiences (such as the ones that underpin fundamental metaphors).

However, it is essential to consider synesthesia in a broader context, recognizing it as a phenomenon that involves cross-activation across diverse sensory or cognitive pathways. As an instance, let us continue with the example derived from Heaney's poem in the previous section, "digging." In the context of the physical act of digging, synesthesia's presence is not directly tied to the concrete act of digging itself. Individuals with synesthesia might experience atypical sensory associations when contemplating digging—such as perceiving colors or tastes linked to the concept of digging. Yet, synesthesia in itself does not inherently form part of the conventional neural network engaged in motor planning or sensory processing for digging, unless we expand our conception of synesthesia to encompass a broader sensory integrative mechanism. In this regard, synesthesia can be considered a cognitive tool that facilitates the connection of brain networks. This perspective aligns with the physical act of digging, where the activation of various regions, including those responsible for motor planning, sensory processing (including tactile and proprioceptive sensations), visual imagery, spatial cognition, and potentially even emotional and contextual associations linked to digging, can be perceived as an amalgamation of brain areas that mimics the characteristics of synesthesia.

In essence, this viewpoint paints synesthesia as an overarching mechanism that facilitates the integration of unrelated areas of the brain. By extending our interpretation of synesthesia to encompass such integrative functions, we can better appreciate its potential role in connecting different brain networks—akin to how the multifaceted process of digging engages various cognitive and sensory domains simultaneously.

The construction of mental representations of fundamental units of experience is deeply connected to sensory engagement. For instance, spatial schemas like balance might involve a trajector-landmark structure to grasp the essence of an object or concept. The use of image schemas, which are perceptual structures, further enriches our cognitive toolkit. These schemas interconnect and stem from recurring patterns of bodily experiences derived from senses like sight, hearing, touch, kinesthetic perception, smell, and even internal sensations like hunger or pain (Grady, 2005: 45).

Primary metaphors often project sensory concepts, frequently identifiable with image schemas, onto non-sensory concepts. The core schematization also finds a connection with synesthesia—a phenomenon that allows us to perceive one sensory experience through another. Synesthesia, acting as a bridge, provides sensory information beyond the concept itself. It can potentially link with the selective attention mechanisms traditionally associated with sensory systems, creating a cohesive and interconnected conceptual system.

The continuous expansion of cognitive schemas shines a light on the intricate interplay that exists among various elements: sensorial experiences, mental representations, metaphorical concepts, and the very bedrock of our cognitive processes. Synesthesia, in this context, stands as a unique conduit—a means to perceive something through another, even when that "something" lacks explicit sensory attributes. By functioning as a provider of sensory experiences that transcend the boundaries of the immediate concept, synesthesia serves as a bridge. This bridge extends from the realm of sensory systems to our conceptual framework, merging the sensory and the conceptual in a harmonious union. Through this bridge, synesthesia connects our cognitive processes with the selective attention mechanisms traditionally linked to sensory systems. In essence, synesthesia becomes a pivotal link that binds our cognitive functions, allowing us to traverse the boundaries between different modes of perception and understanding. This connection illuminates the depth and complexity of how our minds operate, demonstrating the intricate dance between sensory inputs, mental constructs, and the rich tapestry of our cognitive experiences. As synesthesia forges connections beyond the confines of traditional sensory boundaries, it reinforces the unity of our conceptual system, highlighting the remarkable ways in which our cognitive processes enrich our engagement with the world.

2.2.4 Cognition, Primary Metaphors and Emotions

From a cognitive perspective, the intricate interplay between cognition, primary metaphors, and emotions becomes evident (Peña-Cervel and

Ruiz de Mendoza, 2022: 100). Our individual experiences play a pivotal role in shaping both our conceptual frameworks and the overall structure of our minds. Within this framework, the utilization of conceptual metaphor, synesthesia, and blending emerges as vital cognitive tools that are fundamental to our capacity for human understanding. These mechanisms offer a means to cognitively organize and make sense of tangible experiences, exemplified by our ability to convey emotions through expressions like "made me explode" or through the conceptual metaphor ANGER IS HEAT IN A CONTAINER (Gibbs, 1999; Lakoff and Johnson, 1999; Kövecses, 2000; Soriano, 2015). What underlines the potency of these cognitive mechanisms is their direct grounding in our bodily encounters and sensory perceptions.

The connection between primary metaphors (see Figure 4) and emotions lies at the heart of how we understand and express our inner experiences. Primary metaphors are fundamental linguistic and conceptual structures that draw upon our physical and sensory experiences to convey abstract or complex ideas. These metaphors serve as a bridge between our concrete experiences and the more abstract realm of emotions, enabling us to articulate and grasp the intricacies of our feelings.

Emotions are complex psychological states that involve physiological responses, cognitive appraisals, and subjective experiences. These experiences can often be challenging to articulate directly, as they involve a blend of sensations, thoughts, and bodily reactions. Metaphors (see Figure 3) offer a way to capture these nuanced emotional states by mapping them onto more concrete and familiar domains. Substantial individual differences exist in the tendency to experience strong emotional responses, but it has been proven that people who physically respond to music or auditory stimulus with chills have stronger fiber connections between the auditory cortex and emotional processing areas in the brain. This increased connection potentially leads to a heightened ability to experience intense emotions (Sachs et al., 2016). Comparing individual differences in aesthetic response through music or other aesthetic stimuli (such as visual art, dance, poetry or architecture) provides a window onto the interface between the emotion and communication systems in the brain.

Conceptual metaphor (ANGER is a ...)	Metaphorical patterns	N
PRESSURIZED FLUID IN THE BODY-CONTAINER	[anger] rise in X, [anger] wells up in X, contain [anger], vent [anger], [anger] spill-over, outburst of [anger], explode with [anger]	60
FIRE	[anger] burn, flame of [anger], spark [anger], kindle [anger], stoke [anger], blaze with [anger], fume with [anger], [anger] scorch	30
WEAPON	turn/direct/cast [anger] against (/at, /on) Y, target of X's [anger], deflect [anger], [anger] be (sharp) like a knife	29
HOT FLUID	[anger] boil, [anger] simmer, [anger] bubble, [anger] seethe, [anger] sizzle	23
OPPONENT IN A STRUGGLE	fight [anger], conquer [anger], overcome [anger], imprison [anger], [anger] assail X	20
ANIMAL	leash/unleash [anger], rein in [anger], fierce [anger], [anger] roar inside X	13
FORCE OF NATURE	eruption of [anger], storm of [anger], [anger] engulfs X, wave of [anger], [anger] ebbs away, tide of [anger]	10
ILLNESS	spasm of [anger], festering [anger], suffer from [anger], chronic [anger]	6
INSANITY	fit of [anger], beside oneself with [anger]	3

Figure 3. Metaphorical patterns that show how "anger" is conceptualized (taken from Soriano 2015).

As exemplified before, the metaphor ANGER IS HEAT links the physical sensation of heat with the emotional experience of anger. This metaphor allows us to convey the intensity, buildup, and release of anger in a way that is vivid and relatable. Similarly, the metaphor HAPPINESS IS UP connects the idea of upward movement with positive emotions, reflecting how we often associate joy with feelings of elevation, lightness, and positivity.

These primary metaphors provide a shared cognitive framework that allows us to communicate emotions effectively. When we say "I'm on top of the world" to express happiness or "I'm weighed down by sadness" to convey a sense of burden, we are drawing on these metaphors to convey

Metaphors	Examples	Experiential grounding
ANGER IS HEAT	*He's hot under the collar*	We feel hot when experiencing anger because of blood flushing to the surface layers of our skin.
MORE IS UP/LESS IS DOWN	*Prices are going up/down*	We see levels rise and fall as quantity, e.g., of a fluid, increases, or decreases.
AFFECTION IS WARMTH	*She gave me a warm embrace*	We feel warm while being held affectionately.
CHANGE IS MOTION	*She's going from bad to worse*	We tend to correlate certain states with certain locations; e.g., being cool in the shade, warm in bed, safe at home.
IMPORTANT IS BIG	*He's a big wheel in the company*	Large objects exert major forces on other objects and they dominate our visual experience more than small objects.
INTIMACY IS CLOSENESS	*They are very close friends*	When we feel intimate with other people, we tend to become physically close to them.
UNDERSTANDING/ KNOWING IS SEEING	*I see what you mean*	Seeing is a crucial way of getting information.
UNDERSTANDING IS GRASPING	*He was unable to grasp the notion of intersubjectivity*	Touching an object allows us to get information about it.
SIMILARITY IS CLOSENESS	*These two colors are very close*	Often similar objects cluster together (e.g., a flock of birds, the seeds in a piece of fruit, gold nuggets in the bed of a stream, etc.)

Figure 4. Primary metaphors in English (Peña-Cervel and Ruiz de Mendoza, 2022: 100).

complex emotional states in a way that is readily understood by others. In essence, primary metaphors and synesthesia offer a means to bridge the gap between the abstract nature of emotions and the concrete world of our sensorial experiences. By them, we can communicate our emotional landscapes with depth and resonance, allowing others to connect and empathize with our feelings.

As we have seen so far, metaphor operates as the conveyance of information from one realm of meaning to another rendering the abstract tangible. Conversely, synesthesia represents a natural interplay of our mind, manifesting when ordinary stimuli trigger extraordinary conscious experiences (Bretones, 2005). Often, synesthesia has been assimilated within the realm of metaphor in language. But it is not about making the concrete abstract, but rather about experiencing one thing in response to unrelated sensorial information. It involves attributing a quality to something that inherently lacks it, given the distinct ways in which the quality and the item are sensed (e.g., white voices, sweet melodies). In synesthesia, one type of sensory or cognitive input triggers an automatic, involuntary experience in a different sensory or cognitive pathway. Through synesthesia, we grasp and communicate sensorial ideas, simultaneously sharing with others the profound sentiments they evoke within us. Both metaphor and synesthesia play roles in enhancing our understanding and communication, though they involve distinct processes and serve different purposes. While metaphor involves transferring meaning between two different conceptual domains, synesthesia represents a unique sensory interaction where stimulation triggers bodily experiences in different domains.

Take the phrase "boiling sea." The metaphor is initially found in the word "boiling" and the potential for synesthetic qualities arises from the sensory associations evoked in its blend. The word "boiling" is a metaphor in this context. It attributes the quality of "boiling" which is a physical action involving the rapid movement and transformation of a liquid due to heat, to the "sea." The OED defines boiling as the action of heating a liquid to boiling point or of bubbling up under the influence of heat. But we cannot physically boil a sea. These prototypical meaning is overridden by different salient meaning because boiling shows no connection with the sea other than liquidity. While the phrase "boiling see" itself does not explicitly contain synesthetic elements, the metaphor "boiling sea" can activate synesthetic qualities by linking the sensation of "boiling" (visual and tactile) with the concept of a "sea" (visual and auditory). Synesthesia provides the blending of sensory experiences that are not typically associated. In this case, the metaphor might evoke a mental image of a visually turbulent sea, accompanied by an auditory sensation akin to the sound of bubbling or churning water and an emotional state. In summary, the metaphor in "boiling sea" lies in the attribution of the quality of "boiling" to the sea, while the potential for synesthetic qualities arises from the sensory associations evoked by the metaphor, connecting visual and tactile imagery of "boiling" with the concept of a "sea." What is more, synesthesia can also add emotional qualities and thanks to blending the resulting activation can be used to convey a heightened emotional state (EMOTIONS ARE PHYSICAL

STATES OR EMOTION IS HEAT). That implies the subjectification of the sea and its experience of some form of emotional turmoil or agitation similar to the way water boils and bubbles due to heat.

In conclusion, both metaphor and synesthesia make possible the understanding of "boiling see" via blending, including the synesthetic perception of liquid as something physical or emotional, which depending on the context would be felt as a windy-splashy sensation (rough sea) or emotional distress (heated emotions). Blending all this will provide a final stable on-line representation once the frame (generic space) information is introduced. Blending, as depicted in Figure 2, plays a pivotal role in bridging diverse cognitive domains and cognitive tools. Through this process, innovative structures emerge from the amalgamation of concepts, resulting in new and distinct outcomes known as "blends." The notion of *frame* plays a major role here too, as it is defined by cognitive linguistics (Fillmore, 1982, 2006, 2008). Frame goes under a variety of different names in cognitive science, including scene, scenario, model, domain, and even folk theory, just to mention a few, but scholars, such as Kövecses (2019), use frame in a similar way to Fillmore, that is, as any *coherent area of human experience.*

Let us take another example. Heaney in his poem Sunlight (3) writes: "water honeyed in the slung bucket." In it he employs metaphor to describe the water as "honeyed," prototypically conveying a sense of sweetness. The use of "honeyed" also offers synesthetic potential, as it links the idea of sweetness (taste and texture) to the water. The combination of metaphor and potential synesthesia enriches the description, creating a multisensory experience for the reader.

The phrase "water honeyed in the slung bucket" activates a cognitive blend that intricately weaves together metaphor, synesthetic potential, and the frame of sunlight. This blend seamlessly merges different cognitive domains to create a multidimensional sensory experience. It contains:

Metaphoric force:
- The concept of "water honeyed" operates as the base input, utilizing metaphor to attribute the sweetness of honey to the water. This metaphorical mapping enriches the water with the sensory quality of sweetness.

Synesthetic force:
- Within the blend, the synesthetic potential arises within the metaphor itself. The mapping of "honeyed" to the water connects not only the concept of sweetness but also the tactile and viscous qualities of honey. This synesthetic association enhances the sensory richness of the blend.
- The synesthetic potential in "water honeyed" arises from the sensory imagery associated with honey. While the phrase itself does not explicitly convey synesthesia, the metaphorical connection of sweetness to water can create a subtle blending of sensory experiences adding texture. Readers might imagine the feel of honey's texture, the taste of sweetness, and perhaps even a warm, golden visual imagery—all of which can evoke emotional responses tied to sensory comfort and enjoyment.

Emotional Resonance through Blending:
- The blending of metaphor and synesthetic potential in "water honeyed" contributes to an emotional resonance. The fusion of the tactile sensation of honey, the taste of sweetness, and the visual warmth can collectively evoke feelings of comfort, relaxation, and delight. This emotional resonance emerges from the cognitive blend created by the interplay of metaphor and sensory associations.
- While "water honeyed" may not have a direct emotional correlation like the examples involving touch or taste, the metaphorical and synesthetic elements provide a subtle road for emotional resonance by tapping into sensory experiences associated with comfort and pleasure. The blend of metaphor, synesthesia, and potential emotional resonances enriches the imagery and feelings evoked by the phrase.

Frame of Sunlight:
- The blend incorporates the frame in conjunction with "the slung bucket," which positions the entire sensory experience within a specific context. Imagining this scene bathed in sunlight, that is

the typical way in which these elements would heat, adds an extra layer to the blend, introducing visual elements and warmth.

In this cognitive blend, the metaphor, synesthetic potential, and frame of sunlight seamlessly integrate, forming a unified and immersive mental construct. The result is a conceptual fusion that combines taste, texture, visual imagery, and context into a single cohesive experience, engaging multiple cognitive processes and enriching the subject's engagement with the phrase.

2.2.5 *Correlation and Cognitive Condensation*

In the realm of conceptual metaphor theory, conceptual metaphors can find their grounding or "motivation" through essentially two distinct pathways (Grady, 1997, 1999). These pathways are either through resemblance, where the source concept resembles the target concept, or through correlation, where a correlated relationship exists between the source and the target. For instance, the notion of emotion seems very similar to the one of perception, and this resemblance provides an explanation for why emotion can be understood as a form of perception, albeit with differences (see Prinz, 2006). However, this resemblance alone is not enough to account for why the conceptual metaphor EMOTION IS TOUCH in the expression "her words were touching" unmistakably emerges as a metaphorical construct rather than a direct, literal connection. We need a force providing understanding by some kind of cognitive correlation, and that force is synesthesia.

The basis for the metaphor can be traced to shared bodily experiences. The same bodily sensations and organs that come into play in touch, such as skin, temperature changes, and pain, can also be identified in emotions like anger or fear. In this sense, the experiential overlap creates correlations between tactile perceptions and emotional experiences, providing the bodily foundation for the metaphorical linkage (Kövecses, 2019: 15–16). Similarly, in cases involving taste and smell, the metaphorical basis can be traced to shared brain structures. Brain components that contribute to taste and smell, such as the amygdala, also play a role in emotions overall. This correlation establishes a bridge between sensory perceptions and emotions, forming the underlying structure for these metaphors (Kövecses, 2019: 15–16).

In essence, whether it is the metaphor of a "boiling sea" or the blend of a "honeyed water," it can be stated that bodily experiences and brain structures create the intricate web of conceptual information that reveals how our understanding of abstract concepts is deeply rooted in tangible experiences. Differences in variations in the interpretative process exist at the level of the evoked sense given in each case, understanding the instauration of the figurative sense of the construction in the mind. It is precisely there where we see "literality" and "figurativeness," in the different reactions that language evokes, but not by identical cognitive and linguistic mechanisms (Turner, 1998). In any communicative situation we understand the meaning of a word because we are able to infer, interpret, restring or filter the world of possibilities brought by that word through our lexical, episodic and encyclopedic memory by means of a concrete textual processing and certain "psychological" mechanisms (Graesser et al., 1997). From a psycholinguistic point of view, meanings are not static, but they are rebuilt in our mind because they are the result of an act of lexical processing (Clark, 1992; Anderson, 1987). The forms of language carry very few information per se, but they can neat rich relational nets or preexisting networks in the brains of the subjects and cause incredible sequential and parallel activations. Not only in poetic language, but also in language in general, there are occasions when you do not want to make explicit what you actually want to communicate, and you look for a choice that gives the receptors the possibility of inferring the real communicative intention, hidden ideas or covered messages. With this and other purposes we make particular uses of language, and we use what is commonly called figurative language. As mentioned before, this is not the privilege of a few, but it is part of everyday speech (Gibbs, 1994).

It is evident that there is a cognitive-pragmatic relation between the conception of things, the mental states, and the communicative interactions. The observational utterances are interpretations of the world, interpretations of the dates to make them fixed in our world. That makes us affirm that the nature processed by the brain and the senses affect us in our inner self, together with our acquired knowledge through language and the interaction with others. Then, the main problem that we face is that language, due to its own nature, is conceptual. But, at the same time, it is an observable fact that thought sometimes carries within itself emotional, perceptual, or even mistic qualities which give us that "perceived effect" showed on the one hand through the structure and, on the other hand, through what Tsur calls the "regional quality" of a given perceptual object (Tsur, 1992).

The general process that is helping us to integrate all the pieces of the puzzle taking place at different levels, is *cognitive condensation*.

Cognitive condensation is an expression used in the context of cognitive linguistics to describe the process by which complex ideas or concepts are distilled or compressed into more concise and succinct forms, similar to how a gas condenses into a liquid state. There are several related concepts and terms within cognitive science and literary theory that capture the idea of simplifying or condensing complex information or ideas. Here are a few situations in which the general process of condensation is active:

1. Conceptual Compression: This term could refer to the process of reducing complex concepts into more concise and comprehensible forms, like how data compression algorithms condense information for more efficient storage.
2. Schematic Abstraction: This concept involves distilling the essential features of an experience or concept into a simplified mental representation, often in the form of schemas or mental frameworks.
3. Conceptual Synthesis: This term implies the merging or integration of various complex ideas or elements into a unified and simplified concept.
4. Reductive Cognition: Refers to the cognitive process of breaking down complex ideas into simpler components, often to enhance understanding or memory retention.
5. Simplification Heuristics: These are mental shortcuts or strategies that individuals use to simplify complex decision-making processes by focusing on a subset of relevant information.

6. Conceptualization: While not synonymous with condensation, the act of conceptualization involves organizing and structuring complex thoughts or experiences into coherent mental constructs.
7. Summarization: Summarizing involves capturing the main points or essence of a larger body of information in a concise and easily digestible format.
8. Abstraction: Abstraction refers to the process of focusing on the essential characteristics of an object or idea while ignoring irrelevant details, which can lead to a more streamlined and simplified mental representation.

While these terms may not directly mirror cognitive condensation, they encapsulate related ideas and processes of simplification, reduction, and synthesis of complex cognitive content. Depending on the specific context, one of these terms might align more closely with what the concept "cognitive condensation" conveys.

Cognitive condensation provides mental representations, enabled by blending and other cognitive tools like metaphor (Lakoff and Johnson, 1980), synesthesia (Bretones, 2005) and blending (Fauconnier and Turner, 2000) and assumes critical importance for a fundamental cognitive principle that will be explained further in the following chapter: *short story*.

CHAPTER 3

The Iconic Power of the Short Story

3.1 Introduction

The short story can be perceived as a foundational concept within the mind (Turner, 1996). It facilitates communication and renders meaning accessible (Ibáñez, Fernández and Bretones, 2009). At times, to construct intricate frameworks and intricate outcomes, narratives are extended or intertwined. A complex framework in this regard is exemplified by a parable, where one narrative is projected onto another. The underlying cognitive phenomenon making storytelling possible is mental representation (Barsalou, 1999), a highly discerning cognitive process. Mental representation is enabled by cognitive tools such as metaphor (Lakoff and Johnson, 1999), synesthesia (Bretones, 2005) and blending (Fauconnier and Turner, 2000) and assumes critical importance in providing meaning and understanding.

It is believed that the act of storytelling originated through visual narratives, such as those seen in cave paintings and pictograms, before transitioning into oral traditions where stories were passed down from generation to generation verbally,—up to digital media today (Hurlburt and Voas, 2011). Later, the transition to written stories took place. However, the earliest form of mental representation through storytelling was visual, found in paintings within places like caves inhabited by prehistoric communities. Despite this, it is possible that even during that time, certain individuals could invent and narrate stories communicated verbally. It is believed that in those times, the roles of artists, writers, painters, etc., were intertwined with that of shamans or sorcerers who were responsible for providing such forms of "entertainment," although their purpose was not solely for entertainment but rather to convey solid symbolic, mythological, transformative, or educational content. Culture serves as the arena that enables humans to modify their environment and create alternative realities. Humans are seen as deficient beings, not suited to coexist harmoniously with nature, thus necessitating the creation of a second nature to live and survive adequately. This substitutive and artificially adapted world compensates for human organic deficiencies.

The art of storytelling is an inherent part of this second creative nature, stemming from the self-aware constitution of the human animal (Turner, 1996). This human nature, which makes us "open to the world," also causes humans to be bombarded with stimuli, leading to the need to "unload" these stimuli. Consequently, humans feel the constant need to speak, write, narrate, imagine, communicate, and more, in contrast to other animals. There's also an argument that the narrative self has an "evolutionary origin grounded on two pillars: language, without which this narrative self would not exist, and whose emergence profoundly reshapes the human brain, and the reliance on the symbolic and artistic, without which language would not have developed." This perspective suggests that storytelling is a part of our human constitution, a product of biological evolution that has led to the contemporary human as we know it, the homo sapiens or "wise man." Moreover, storytelling would be a byproduct or epiphenomenon of our capacity for—and need to—communicate with one another, given our social nature as communal animals always in need of social interaction. Nowadays, new technologies, particularly the internet, have transformed how we tell stories. Starting around the year 2000 with the proliferation of mobile phones and the use of SMS, linguistic abbreviations in written formats, emojis, etc. up to the present day where gifs and memes have become powerful communicative vehicles in our everyday lives (see Hurlburt and Voas, 2011). We have micro fiction, flash fiction, haikus and others.

The short story plays a crucial role in capturing and conveying the essence of human experiences, ideas, and emotions. It is the paramount example of cognitive condensation. Just as storytelling has evolved from visual narratives to written and digital forms, the short story remains a potent medium for encapsulating the complexity of human existence within a concise format. Its ability to condense intricate narratives, character development, and thematic exploration into a brief space resonates with the human need for efficient communication and connection. Through the short story, individual can harness the power of language and symbolism to create microcosms of meaning, echoing our fundamental inclination to convey, share, and make sense of the multifaceted world around us. As technology advances, the short story continues to adapt, finding new ways to resonate with contemporary readers while maintaining its timeless ability to encapsulate the human experience.

3.2 The Short Story as Basic Principle of Mind

The story is a basic principle of mind, and every level of our experience is interpreted by means of cognitive devices (for instance, metaphor, metonymy, synesthesia, blending) which have cognitive and biological grounds (Turner, 1996; Ibáñez-Ibáñez, Fernández Sánchez and Bretones Callejas, 2007).

Short stories can be conceived as cognitive devices because they engage the reader's imagination and encourage them to think critically and creatively about the world. In many ways, reading a short story is like solving a puzzle or completing a mental exercise. The reader is presented with a series of clues and must use their analytical skills to piece together the meaning of the story. This process of deciphering meaning can help to sharpen the reader's cognitive abilities and enhance their understanding of the world around them.

Moreover, short stories often deal with complex and nuanced themes, such as love, loss, and human nature, that require the reader to think deeply and critically about the human experience. By grappling with these themes, the reader can develop a more nuanced and sophisticated understanding of the world and their place in it.

In this sense, short stories can be seen as a form of cognitive training or exercise that helps to stimulate the mind and promote intellectual growth. They encourage readers to think creatively and flexibly, and to develop their ability to analyze, interpret, and understand complex texts and ideas.

Making sense of short stories is different from long narratives because the brevity of the form makes readers more involved cognitively, contributing input from their personal experience and their cultural knowledge when responding to the gaps and absences in the text (Brosch, 2013, 2015, 2017, 2018 a & b). Both short stories and poetry focus on brevity and conciseness, use similar narrative techniques and have the ability to evoke powerful emotions. When facing them, readers are required cognitive involvement, which may be defined as a concern with the functional information content of a communication, and affective involvement (Stansfield and Bruce, 2014), defined as a concern with the emotional and value expressive content of a communication. They can be seen as a form of cognitive stimulation that engages the reader's mind and promotes intellectual growth. They encourage readers to think creatively and flexibly, and to develop their ability to analyze, interpret, and understand complex texts and ideas.

Short stories and poetry share similarities, particularly in their use of language and literary devices to create an emotional impact on the reader. Both forms of literature often rely on vivid imagery, sensory details, and figurative language to convey a message or tell a story. One significant parallelism between short stories and poetry is their focus on brevity and conciseness. Both forms of literature strive to convey their message in a compact form, utilizing carefully chosen words and evocative imagery to create a powerful impact on the reader. In this sense, a well-crafted short story can have a similar emotional resonance as that of a poem. Another parallelism between the two is the use of narrative techniques to create a sense of coherence and structure. While poems are characteristically more condensed and free-flowing than short stories, both forms use narrative techniques like plot, characterization, and setting to create a compelling story or message.

The concept of a poem as a short story is a fascinating approach that blurs the traditional boundaries between poetry and prose narrative. While poetry and short stories are distinct literary forms, they share common elements in their exploration of themes, characters, emotions, and human experiences. Viewing a poem as a short story allows for a deeper appreciation of the narrative and storytelling aspects present in both forms.

Here are some key considerations when approaching a poem as a short story:

1. Narrative Elements: Just like a short story, a poem can contain narrative elements such as characters, settings, conflicts, and resolutions. These elements create a sense of progression and engage readers in a narrative journey.
2. Imagery and Description: Poems often use vivid imagery and descriptive language to evoke emotions and paint a picture in the reader's mind. These elements can create a rich visual and sensory experience similar to what is found in short stories.
3. Character Development: While poems might not have the same space as short stories to extensively develop characters, they can still provide glimpses into the thoughts, emotions, and experiences of characters. Poetic techniques like interior monologue or persona can help create a sense of character depth.
4. Themes and Emotions: Both poems and short stories explore universal themes and emotions that resonate with readers. Whether it is love, loss, identity, or social issues, the emotional impact of a poem can be as powerful as that of a short story.
5. Narrative Arc: Some poems have a discernible narrative arc, where they introduce a situation or conflict, build tension, and provide resolution. This structure is reminiscent of the classic arc found in short stories.
6. Economy of Language: Poets often work with limited words to convey layered meanings. This economy of language can be compared to the concise nature of short stories, where every word carries weight.
7. Open to Interpretation: Both poems and short stories leave room for interpretation, inviting readers to engage actively with the text. The brevity of poems, like short stories, can stimulate readers' imagination and critical thinking.
8. Different Forms of Poetry: Various forms of poetry, such as narrative poetry or dramatic monologues, lend themselves more

naturally to the concept of a poem as a short story due to their focus on storytelling.

Ultimately, the idea of viewing a poem as a short story emphasizes the narrative potential of poetry. It encourages readers to approach poems with a storytelling lens and highlights the versatility of language and form in expressing the complexities of human experiences.

Each short story provides a structure as it follows (see Zwaan, Magliano and Graesser, 1995: 192; Herman, 2005: 43):

1. the time frame in which it occurs (TIME)
2. the spatial region in which it occurs (GROUND)
3. the protagonist (or protagonists) it involves (FIGURE)
4. its causal status with regard to the prior event (EVENT)
5. its relatedness to a protagonist's goals (GOAL).

From there the story can be updated or re-indexed using blending (Faucconier and Turner, 2002). This story schema provides at least two benefits. First, to delineate a scene with quick gestures. Second, in general terms the schema allows authors to call attention to departures from what is considered canonically as the norm (Herman, 2005: 41).

We can extrapolate these similarities between short stories and poetry to the work of Seamus Heaney, known for his use of vivid imagery and powerful language to explore themes related to Irish culture, history, and identity. Given his work, his skillful use of language and his exploration of various themes, it is possible that Heaney might have appreciated the idea posed in this book of viewing a poem as a short story, especially if it allowed for a richer exploration of characters, emotions, and narrative elements within the constraints of a poetic form. We shall see it in depth in next section. Heaney was known for pushing the boundaries of traditional poetic conventions, experimenting with various forms and styles and if asked about the concept of a poem as a short story, Heaney might have expressed that both forms share a common goal: to engage readers, evoke emotions, and offer insights into the human condition and even though he wrote mainly poetry and essays, his work shares parallels with short stories in its ability to convey a narrative or tell a story through the use of vivid imagery, characterization, and setting. Many of Heaney's poems depict scenes from rural life in Ireland, drawing on his own experiences growing up on a farm in County Derry. Through his use of rich sensory details and evocative language, Heaney is able to create a vivid picture of the landscapes, people, and traditions of Ireland, and to explore complex situations reflecting identity, belonging, and the relationship between past and present.

In summary, Heaney's poetry shares many of the same narrative and thematic elements as short stories, including its use of vivid imagery, characterization, and setting to convey a story or message. However, Heaney's poetry employs sometimes a nonlinear structure, allowing for multiple stories or perspectives to be woven together in a single poem. This can create a sense of complexity and depth, as well as a sense of the interconnectedness of diverse aspects of Irish culture and history. For example, in his poem "Digging," Heaney weaves together his memories of his father's work as a potato farmer, his own identity as a poet, and his relationship to the Irish landscape and literary tradition. The result is a multifaceted exploration of themes related to family, work, identity, and artistic creation.

3.3 Cognitive, Affective and Cultural Dimensions in Short Story

Several researchers and scholars have made significant contributions to the study of cognitive processes and affective involvement in reading and understanding literary texts. Some of these researchers have explored aspects of cognitive involvement, comprehension, and interpretation in literary contexts, such as Oatley (2016), Zunshine (2015) or Miall and Kuiken (2002). Another researcher known for his contributions to the field of cognitive linguistics, story and cross-cultural studies of language is Dan Slobin with his famous research project "Frog Stories" focusing on cross-linguistic and cross-cultural differences in narrative structure,— particularly how different languages and cultures convey events, actions, and relationships in storytelling (Slobin, 2004). While his work is not centered on short stories in the literary sense, it does have implications for understanding how narratives are constructed and conveyed across cultures. Slobin's research has explored the role of Theory of Mind (the ability to understand and attribute mental states to others) in narrative comprehension. He has investigated how short narratives provide insight into characters' thoughts, emotions, and intentions, contributing to the broader understanding of cognitive and emotional engagement in storytelling.

Heaney's poem "Digging" (1966), which has been used along this book as a master example of iconicity, could be reviewed using a cross-cultural and cognitive approach inspired by Dan Slobin's "Frog Stories" research, examining how cultural and cognitive factors influence the narrative structure, language use, and cognitive processes evoked by the poem. All in all, exploring how "Digging" reflects cognitive universals and cultural variations. This is how we could approach the poem:

- Narrative Structure and Event Sequencing: The narrative structure of "Digging" follows a reflective and introspective pattern. The speaker describes the act of digging, connects it to his family's history of manual labor, and reflects on his personal choice to pursue writing instead. In "Digging," the narrative structure centers on the speaker's reflection on the act of digging and its personal significance. The narrative unfolds through the speaker's memories and observations, creating a reflective and introspective atmosphere. See some example lines from "Digging":

    > Between my finger and my thumb
    > The squat pen rests; snug as a gun.
    > Under my window, a clean rasping sound
    > When the spade sinks into gravelly ground:
    > My father, digging. I look down
    > Till his straining rump among the flowerbeds
    > Bends low, comes up twenty years away

> Stooping in rhythm through potato drills
> Where he was digging.

- Cultural Embedding and Interpretation: "Digging" embeds cultural elements related to family heritage and labor. The speaker's reflection on his father's manual labor and his own choice of a different path reflects cultural values and generational transitions.
- Language and Cognitive Processing: The poem's language evokes sensory imagery, such as "clean rasping sound" and "squat pen rests." Readers engage in mental imagery as they visualize the scenes described, demonstrating how language influences cognitive involvement.
- Theory of Mind and Character Perspectives: Readers engage in Theory of Mind by inferring the speaker's emotions and thoughts, as well as his father's experiences. The speaker's empathy for his father's labor and his own aspirations invokes readers' cognitive and emotional engagement.
- Narrative Variation and Cultural Expression: "Digging" reflects a cultural narrative of familial heritage and choice. It explores the tension between tradition and individuality, which resonates with broader cultural narratives of self-identity and heritage.
- Reader Response and Cognitive Engagement: Readers from different cultural backgrounds might engage with the poem differently. Those with similar cultural experiences may connect deeply with the themes of heritage and choice, while readers from other cultures may engage with the universal themes of self-discovery and identity.
- Emotional Resonance and Affective Involvement: The poem's emotional resonance is achieved through its exploration of family legacy and personal aspirations. Readers' affective responses are shaped by their own experiences, cultural perspectives, and cognitive processes.
- Cultural and linguistic factors can influence how events are sequenced, connected, and conveyed in narratives. Similarities and differences in narrative structure provide insights into cognitive and cultural patterns of storytelling.

Incorporating these research elements into the analysis of "Digging" offers a unique perspective on the poem's cognitive, affective and cultural dimensions providing its iconic power. By applying Slobin's cross-cultural approach, we can illuminate how the poem's narrative structure, language, and themes intersect with readers' cognitive involvement and cultural contexts.

3.4　The Iconic Power of the Short Story in Heaney

The iconic power of a short story refers to its ability to convey universal themes and ideas that resonate with readers across time and cultures. A short story that possesses iconic power has the capacity to capture the human condition in a way that is both timeless and immediately recognizable, making it a work that endures and remains relevant to new generations of readers. In the case of short stories, iconic power can be seen in works like Edgar Allan Poe's *The Tell-Tale Heart* (1843), which has become an enduring emblem of psychological horror, or James Joyce's *The Dead* (1914), which explores universal themes of love, loss, and mortality. In the case of poetry, iconic power refers also to its ability to capture the essence of a particular moment or experience in a way that is both timeless and universal. This power comes from the use of language and imagery to create a lasting impression on the reader, invoking emotions and ideas that go beyond the immediate context of the poem.

The concept of iconic power in poetry has been explored by several scholars and critics. Harold Bloom, in his book *The Anxiety of Influence* (1997), discusses the idea of strong poetry that has the power to shape and influence future poets. T. S. Eliot, in his essay *Tradition and the Individual Talent* (1920), argues that iconic poetry transcends its historical moment to speak to larger human truths. More recent scholars, such as Helen Vendler and Marjorie Perloff, have also written extensively on the concept of iconic power in poetry. Vendler, in her book *The Breaking of Style* (1995), examines how poetic form and language can create a sense of iconic power that transcends individual poems. Perloff, in her book *Unoriginal Genius* (2010), explores how the use of intertextuality in contemporary literature can create a sense of iconic power by connecting poems to larger cultural and literary traditions (Guerra, 2019; Pereira, 2019).

Heaney's work often transcend historic moments drawing on his childhood memories of rural Ireland, and his vivid descriptions of landscapes, animals, and natural phenomena evoke a sense of wonder and awe that is both immediate and enduring. Take the case of this short biographic description which tells the reader a whole story about him (Heaney, 1988: 3):

> In 1939, the year that Patrick Kavanagh arrived in Dublin, an aunt of mine planted a chestnut in a jam jar. When it began to sprout she broke the jar, made a hole and transplanted the thing under a hedge in front of the house. Over the years, the seedling shot up into a young tree that rose taller and taller above the boxwood hedge. And over the years I came to identify my own life with the life of the chestnut tree.
>
> This was because everybody remembered and constantly repeated the fact that it had been planted the year I was born; also because I was something of a favourite with that particular aunt, so her affection came to be symbolized in the tree; and also perhaps because the chestnut was the one significant thing that grew as I grew. The rest of the trees and hedges round the house were all mature and appeared therefore like given features of the world: the chestnut tree, on the other hand, was young and was watched in much the same way as the other children and myself were watched and commented upon, fondly, frankly and unrelentingly.
>
> When I was in my early teens, the family moved away from that house and the new owners of the place eventually cut down every tree around the yard and the lane and the garden, including the chestnut tree. We deplored that, of course, but life went on.

After reading this, we can highlight the iconic power of one specific figure, the one of the chestnut tree. That image shows the process of being nurtured, cherished and finally removed, parallel to the story of any loved, cherished and finally unrooted person.

The concept of iconic power in poetry is a complex and multifaceted one, ingrained in the ability of language and imagery to create lasting impressions on the reader. Its exploration has been a key focus of literary scholarship and criticism for many years and continues to be a source of inspiration and debate for poets and readers alike. But in the context of this book, iconic power is studied within a broader framework, as it deepens into the characterization of the short story as a fundamental aspect of the mind, encompassing its significant attributes, and emphasizes the necessity for in-depth exploration.

Regarding other fields, Susan Sontag, in her book *On Photography* (1977), uses iconic power to describe the emotional and psychological impact of certain photographs. She argues that some photographs have the ability to become cultural icons or symbols that evoke strong emotional and cultural associations, suggesting that the iconic power of a photograph is not necessarily related to the subject matter or content of the image, but rather to the way the image is composed and presented. She argues that photographs with strong iconic power often have a simple and direct composition, with clear lines and contrasts that create a striking visual impact. Sontag also suggests that the iconic power of a photograph can be influenced by its historical and cultural context. Photographs that capture significant historical events or cultural moments may become powerful symbols of those events or moments and may be used to evoke a wide range of emotional and cultural associations. Sontag's concept of iconic power suggests that certain cultural artifacts, including photographs, have the ability to become powerful symbols that evoke strong emotional and cultural associations, and that the composition and context of these artifacts can play an important role in shaping their impact and meaning. Although the concept of *iconic power* is not a fixed or objective measure and can vary depending on the individual reader's interpretation and response to the artifact in question, it could easily be stated that it implies endurance across time and cultures, remaining relevant and resonant with readers for generations. The stories told in the text above or in poems are like photographs. They stay in our retina and remain as full pictures.

The idea that stories told in poems are like photographs, staying in our memory as vivid images, is a metaphorical concept traditionally suggested by literary criticism through the analysis of imagery, but poetry, as everyday language, uses descriptive language to create mental pictures all the time. The connection between poetry, everyday language, and mental representations aligns with the concepts explored in cognitive science, particularly as described by Lawrence Barsalou's theory of perceptual symbol systems (2008). Barsalou's theory suggests that cognition involves the use of perceptual and sensory information to form mental representations of concepts and experiences. In the context of poetry, this theory can help explain how language creates vivid mental pictures and engages readers' sensory and cognitive processes. When writers use everyday language to describe scenes, emotions, or experiences, they tap into readers' existing mental representations. Here's how poetry aligns with Barsalou's theory and cognitive science:

1. Embodied Simulation: According to Barsalou's theory, mental representations are not abstract symbols but are grounded in perceptual and sensory experiences. When a poet uses descriptive language, readers simulate sensory experiences in their minds. For example, a poem describing a sunlit forest might trigger mental simulations of the visual scene, sounds of rustling leaves, and the feeling of warmth.
2. Conceptual Blending: Barsalou's theory emphasizes the blending of perceptual and sensory information to form concepts. Poetry often employs metaphor and analogy, which involve blending different domains of experience to create new meanings. These conceptual blends help readers create mental images by combining familiar sensory elements.
3. Activation of Sensory Cortex: Reading descriptive poetry activates regions of the brain associated with sensory experiences. As readers engage with vivid language, their brains simulate sensory and perceptual details, resulting in a richer and more immersive understanding of the text.
4. Immersive Experience: Effective poetry encourages readers to mentally simulate the experiences described in the text. By triggering sensory and perceptual mental representations, readers become actively engaged in creating and experiencing the mental pictures the poet conveys.
5. Subjective Experience: Barsalou's theory acknowledges the subjective nature of mental representations. Different readers might have slightly different mental simulations based on their personal experiences and memories. This uniqueness contributes to the individual and personal experience of reading poetry.

In summary, the use of everyday language in poetry aligns with cognitive performance because it activates readers' sensory and perceptual systems to create mental representations. This allows poets to evoke vivid mental pictures and emotions in readers' minds, making the reading experience more immersive and engaging. As readers process the descriptive language, their brains simulate sensory experiences, enabling them to construct a rich and personalized understanding of the poem.

The use of specific and detailed adjectives, adverbs, nouns, and verbs to paint a clear picture in the reader's mind. Instead of saying "a beautiful flower," you could describe it as "a delicate, crimson rose." Engage multiple senses by describing how something looks, sounds, smells, tastes, or feels. This sensory information helps readers immerse themselves in the experience. For instance, "The air was heavy with the scent of blooming jasmine, and the birds sang sweet melodies" instead of directly stating information, shows it through actions, dialog, or descriptions. This allows readers to infer and visualize the details. For instance, instead of saying "He was sad," you could write "His shoulders slumped, and his eyes grew misty." The use dynamic verbs and action-oriented language to engage readers in the unfolding events helps them imagine the sequence of actions and emotions. It connects emotions to visual cues to deepen the reader's understanding of a character's feelings and allows readers to form rich mental images and immerse themselves in the world created.

Susan Sontag's concept of iconic power and Chris Sinha's concept of cognitive artifacts both explore the ways in which cultural artifacts can shape our perceptions and understanding of the world around us. According to Sinha (2009, 2015), cognitive artifacts are objects or tools that we use to extend our cognitive abilities and interact with the world. They are designed to shape our thinking and help us navigate complex environments. Examples of cognitive artifacts include maps, diagrams, and even language itself. Similarly, Sontag's concept of iconic power suggests that cultural artifacts like photographs can shape our understanding of the world by evoking strong emotional and cultural associations. Photographs, like other cultural artifacts, can become symbols that help us interpret and make sense of the world around us. In both cases, the power of these artifacts comes from their ability to shape our perceptions and understanding of the world.

Cognitive artifacts are designed to enhance our cognitive abilities, while cultural artifacts like photographs and literature are designed to evoke emotional and cultural associations that shape our understanding of the world. Overall, the concepts of cognitive artifacts and iconic power offer different perspectives on the ways in which cultural artifacts can shape our perceptions and understanding of the world, but both suggest that these artifacts play an important role in how we make sense of our experiences.

In Heaney's poem "Digging" (1966) the pen becomes an artifact that can be seen as an icon of the act of writing and the power of language. The pen is also associated with the act of digging and physical labor, suggesting a connection between the physical and intellectual work of creating art. The poem itself can also be seen as a cultural artifact with its own iconic power, as it has become a widely read and studied work of poetry that has had a significant impact on the field of literature. In this sense, one could argue that the pen in "Digging" and the poem itself both have a certain level of iconic power as cultural artifacts that evoke strong emotional and intellectual associations for readers.

One of the strongest iconic powers in Heaney's poetry is its ability to capture the complexities and contradictions of identity and history in everyday stories. Through his use of language, imagery, and historical references, Heaney is able to convey the unique cultural and political landscape of Ireland, while also connecting this landscape to broader human experiences. He explores his own relationship to his family's farming traditions, using the metaphor of digging to explore the connections between the past and the present (lines 1–9):

> Between my finger and my thumb
> The squat pen rests; snug as a gun.
> Under my window, a clean rasping sound
> When the spade sinks into gravelly ground:
> My father, digging. I look down
> Till his straining rump among the flowerbeds
> Bends low, comes up twenty years away
> Stooping in rhythm through potato drills
> Where he was digging.

Through his use of language and imagery, Heaney is able to connect the act of digging with broader themes of labor, memory, and identity, evoking the unique cultural landscape of Ireland while also exploring the human experiences that underlie this landscape. In this way, the iconic power of Seamus Heaney's poetry lies in its ability to convey the specificity of Irish history and culture while also evoking broader human experiences that resonate with readers across cultural and national boundaries. "Digging" (1966) describes the work of his father and grandfather as farmers, and reflects on the relationship between the land, the body, and the imagination. Through his use of rich imagery and sensory detail, Heaney creates a vivid portrait of his family's history and cultural heritage, while also exploring the deeper themes of identity, creativity, and connection (lines 28–31).

> But I've no spade to follow men like them.
> Between my finger and my thumb
> The squat pen rests.
> I'll dig with it.

We can analyze the utterance "dig with my pen" in the poem's context and see the basic conceptual metaphor activated to make understanding possible: IDEAS ARE BURIED TREASURES. Conceptual Metaphor Theory, which suggests that abstract concepts are often understood and expressed through more concrete and experiential concepts, allows us the iconic representation of a pen that has a main function, the act of digging. In this context we easily identify the target domain, that is, the abstract concept conveyed, which is "ideas." The source domain is the more concrete and experiential concept that is used to understand the target domain. In this case, the source domain is "buried treasures." The metaphorical mapping would work as follows:

- Ideas (Target or Input 2) are understood in terms of Buried Treasures (Source or Input 1).

Here's why the "Ideas are Buried Treasures" metaphor is activated in the sentence "I'll dig with my pen":

1. Association with Unearthing or Discovery: The act of digging is associated with uncovering something hidden or buried beneath the surface. Similarly, when you use your pen to write or express ideas, you are metaphorically "unearthing" or "discovering" those ideas and bringing them to the surface.
2. Value and Effort: Buried treasures are valuable and often require effort to find and retrieve. Similarly, when you use the word "dig" to describe writing with your pen, you suggest that the act of generating ideas requires effort and has value.
3. Metaphorical Use: The use of the word "dig" in the context of writing creates a linguistic bridge between the concrete action of physically digging and the more abstract action of expressing ideas through writing. This linguistic link activates the metaphor and helps convey the idea of exploring and uncovering ideas.

Conceptual metaphors like IDEAS ARE BURIED TREASURES allow us to understand and communicate complex and abstract concepts by grounding them in more familiar and concrete experiences. In this case, the metaphor enriches the meaning of the sentence "I dig with my squat pen," suggesting a deeper engagement with the act of writing and the process of bringing ideas to light. But applying blending theory to the sentence, we can see the process of conceptual integration that allows the access and combination of distinct mental spaces to create a new conceptual space that captures its iconic strength, provided by the metaphorical link between digging and writing. The conceptual integration approach, also called *blending theory*, highlights the cognitive mechanisms that allow us to make sense of complex metaphors and create richer interpretations of language and mental picture (Turner and Fauconnier, 1995, 1996, 1997). While the metaphorical spaces integrate through mapping providing first the connection of Input Spaces 1 and 2, distinct mental spaces with their own elements and structure (MS1 involves digging and unearthing, while MS2 involves writing and expressing ideas), the creation of a Generic Space (GS) where elements from both input spaces are integrated representing a blended scenario where the physical act of digging is metaphorically linked to the act of writing with a pen and there is Selective Projection creating emergent structure in the Generic Space. This structure combines the action of digging with the act of writing, highlighting the effortful and valuable nature of expressing ideas. Through the blending process, (1) readers infer a connection between digging and writing, allowing to see the act of writing as a metaphorical form of unearthing ideas and (2) the meaning of the sentence "I dig with my pen" enriches by conveying the idea that the process of writing involves a deep engagement, similar to the effort and value associated with uncovering buried treasures. The emergent structure in the blend combines the act of writing with the concept of a squat person ready to uncover buried treasures.

The blend creates an iconic representation that combines elements from physical action (digging) and creative expression (writing), being the pen the cultural artifact that becomes a metaphorical tool for "digging" into the mind to discover ideas. The blend creates a coherent and meaningful mental representation of the act of writing as an exploratory process that uncovers and reveals ideas, much like digging unearths buried treasures.

Blending conveys the story that writing is a form of creative excavation, where the pen becomes a metaphorical tool for unearthing and bringing to light meaningful insights and thoughts. It allows us to mentally visualize the physical action of digging while simultaneously understanding its metaphorical counterpart in writing. Blending helps us understand the iconic power of the story and see how language and metaphor operate, creating novel and imaginative connections between seemingly unrelated concepts.

Iconic representations sometimes evolve into symbolic representations, especially when they become widely recognized and associated with abstract concepts or meanings beyond their initial concrete referents. The transition from iconic to symbolic representation occurs when the original concrete connection between the signifier (the representation) and the signified (the meaning) becomes more abstract and conventional.

Here's how this transition can take place:

1. Iconic Representation: An iconic representation is a direct resemblance or similarity between the signifier and the signified. It relies on a recognizable and perceptible connection between the

two. For example, a simple drawing of a person can be an iconic representation of an actual person.
2. Symbolic Representation: A symbolic representation involves a conventionally established relationship between the signifier and the signified. The connection between the two is not based on a direct resemblance but on shared cultural understanding or agreement. Symbols often carry broader and abstract meanings, normally in graphic ways. For instance, a red heart symbolizes love, even though it doesn't resemble an actual human heart. Graphic symbols, like in the example given, are considered to be even better remembered than words, because they offer a straightforward visual referent for abstract concepts that are otherwise unlikely to be spontaneously imaged. They concretize abstract concepts and, thanks to this, they outperform words in memory tests (see Roberts, MacLeod and Fernandes, 2023).

The transition from iconic to symbolic representation occurs as people begin to associate the original concrete representation with broader and more abstract meanings. Over time, the connection between the representation and its original concrete referent weakens, and the representation becomes a cultural symbol with a shared and conventionalized meaning. The transition from iconic to symbolic representation is influenced by cultural context, shared understanding, and historical factors. As people collectively attach new meanings to a representation, it can acquire symbolic significance beyond its initial concrete resemblance. The evolution of an iconic representation into a symbol is a gradual and complex process influenced by factors such as linguistic usage, cultural trends, and shared interpretations. Not all iconic representations necessarily become symbols, but under the right conditions, an iconic representation like "pen-digging" could potentially develop into a meaningful symbol with broader and more abstract connotations.

Initially, the phrase "dig with the pen" contains an iconic representation where the act of writing with a pen is metaphorically linked to the action of digging. The representation directly resembles the idea of exploration and discovery through writing. If the phrase "dig with the pen" gains widespread recognition and usage, people may start associating it not only with the physical act of writing but also with the broader concept of creative exploration, uncovering ideas, and expressing oneself. The transition to a symbol would depend on cultural factors, the context in which the phrase is used, and whether it resonates with a shared understanding among a community of speakers or writers. If the phrase becomes associated with deeper philosophical or literary concepts, it might start to carry symbolic weight beyond its initial concrete connection. In a rural environment such as Ireland where ideas had a deep impact, it is probable that this icon became soon a symbol, evoking various associations depending on context and cultural interpretations. Here are some symbolic associations commonly linked to the concept of digging:

1. Exploration and Discovery: Digging is often associated with the idea of uncovering hidden or buried things. Symbolically, it can represent the act of exploring new ideas, knowledge, or insights, and the process of discovering previously unknown aspects of oneself or the world.
2. Growth and Transformation: Just as digging prepares the ground for planting, it can symbolize the preparation and effort required for personal or spiritual growth. The act of digging can be seen as a metaphor for breaking through barriers and cultivating change.
3. Effort and Persistence: Digging requires physical effort and determination. Symbolically, it can represent the virtues of hard work, patience, and perseverance in achieving one's goals.
4. Unearthing the Past: Digging can unearth artifacts from the past. Symbolically, it can represent going into one's personal history, memories, or cultural heritage, as well as the process of confronting and addressing unresolved issues.
5. Burial and Release: While digging is often associated with uncovering, it can also symbolize the act of burying or letting go. Symbolically, it may represent the process of leaving behind old habits, negative emotions, or past experiences.

6. Inner Exploration: Digging can be metaphorically applied to inner exploration, representing the process of self-discovery, introspection, and understanding one's emotions and motivations.
7. Catharsis and Cleansing: Digging can be seen as a way to clear away debris and create a fresh start. Symbolically, it may represent the cathartic process of releasing emotional burdens and purging negative influences.

Some of this symbolic associations could be found in the full poem:

1. Exploration and Discovery: In "Digging," the act of digging symbolizes the speaker's exploration of his family's history and heritage. He describes his father and grandfather as skilled diggers, connecting the act of digging to a tradition of manual labor and exploration of the earth. The act of holding the pen represents the speaker's exploration and discovery of his own identity and family history through writing (e.g., "Between my finger and my thumb The squat pen rests; snug as a gun.").
2. Growth and Transformation: While the theme of growth and transformation may not be explicitly addressed in the poem, the speaker's reflection on his own role as a writer can be seen as a form of personal and creative growth, a transformation from the labor of the past to the art of the present. The speaker acknowledges the transformation from a laborer like his father and grandfather to a writer, using a pen as his tool of growth (e.g. "By God, the old man could handle a spade. Just like his old man." Or, for example, "But I've no spade to follow men like them.").
3. Effort and Persistence: The poem emphasizes the effort and persistence required for manual labor, as seen in the descriptions of the digging process. The speaker contrasts his own writing efforts with his family's physical labor, highlighting the different forms of dedication and perseverance (e.g., "Nicking and slicing neatly, heaving sods Over his shoulder, going down and down For the good turf.").

4. Unearthing the Past: The poem revolves around the idea of unearthing the past, both in terms of the family's history of digging and the speaker's exploration of his roots. The act of digging serves as a metaphor for uncovering and understanding the past (e.g., "Till his straining rump among the flowerbeds Bends low, comes up twenty years away Stooping in rhythm through potato drills").
5. Burial and Release: While burial and release are not explicit themes, the act of digging can be seen as both a burial of the past and a release of the memories and stories that are connected to the labor of digging (e.g., "The cold smell of potato mould, the squelch and slap Of soggy peat, the curt cuts of an edge Through living roots awaken in my head.").
6. Inner Exploration: The speaker engages in a form of inner exploration as he reflects on his identity and his connection to his family's history. His introspective examination serves as a metaphorical form of digging into his own thoughts and emotions (e.g., "The squat pen rests; snug as a gun. Under my window, a clean rasping sound When the spade sinks into gravelly ground.").
7. Catharsis and Cleansing: The cathartic aspect of digging is implied in the poem's contemplation of the speaker's personal journey. The act of writing becomes a way for the speaker to cleanse and make sense of his own experiences and heritage (e.g. "The squat pen rests; I'll dig with it.").

In "Digging," Seamus Heaney uses the act of digging as a powerful symbol that encapsulates various layers of meaning, including the exploration of the past, the connection to heritage, and the speaker's introspective journey. While not all the mentioned symbols may be directly addressed in the poem, the overarching themes and imagery align with the symbolic associations mentioned.

Digging is often associated with the idea of uncovering hidden or buried things. Symbolically, it can represent the act of exploring new ideas, knowledge, or insights, and the process of discovering previously unknown aspects of oneself or the world.

The iconic power of short story in poetry resides then in its ability to become a symbol or representation of a particular idea, emotion, or experience. It is the ability of a short literary work to transcend the specific and to speak to broader human themes and concerns. The strongest iconic power of Seamus Heaney's poetry is its ability to connect the specific experiences of Irish history and culture with universal themes of human experience and emotion. Heaney's poetry often draws on the landscapes, language, and traditions of Ireland, and many of his poems explore the complex history of the country and its people. However, Heaney's work is not limited to a specific time or place, and his poetry has a universal quality that speaks to human experiences of love, loss, longing, and joy. Heaney's strongest iconic power is his ability to create a sense of connection between the particular and the universal, between the specific experiences of his own life and the broader themes of human existence.

CHAPTER 4

Story, Metaphor and the Cognitive Phenomenon

4.1 Story, Metaphoric Understanding and Schemas

This book and the approach that it proposes argue for the importance of short stories not only as part of literature, but also as a literary capacity indispensable to human cognition (Turner, 1996). Most of our experience, knowledge, and thinking is organized as stories (Herman, 2003: 2) and beyond it is parable, being defined by the OED as the expression of one story through another. As C. S. Lewis (1982, 2013) observed, that does not belong merely to literary criticism but to mind in general. These are precisely the aims of cognitive studies, to analyze the basic principles of the mind and find the characteristics of the whole formed by language, thought and mind.

You tell stories when you explain to your friend that things *went* well in your trip to Rome, when you explain to your students that the subject *locates* before the verb in affirmative sentences, when you tell the doctor that you feel *pins and needles* when you swallow, and you receive stories when, for example, the doctor explains to you that you are *fighting* a virus. All these stories are everyday stories which help us to come to terms with reality and they show how most of our experience, knowledge, and thinking is organized as stories. But in the examples given before, a trip cannot *go* unless it is conceptualized as an animated object, the subject of a sentence does not *locate* unless it is conceptualized as an animate object as well, we do not feel actual *needles* but a sore throat when we have a cold, and finally our body does not *fight* a battle but recovers from an illness. So that, those stories are possible thanks to specific cognitive mechanisms or structures that help us conceptualize things in different terms. Thanks to linguistic metaphors some conceptual projection is expressed with words. There is an infinity of expressions at the level of concrete words, but we can affirm that they derive mainly from a few basic metaphors at a conceptual level (Lakoff and Johnson, 1980; Lakoff and Turner, 1989).

Most of our normal conceptual system is structured metaphorically and that means that most concepts are partially understood in terms of other concepts. The mentioned conceptual system will be defined not only by internal representations according to the speaker's vision of the world, but also by his or her experience; physical, emotional, mental, cultural or any other. That conceptual system is shared by the members of a specific culture, the Occidental in our case. Thus, metaphor is not just a discursive figure found in poetry, but as a cognitive process by means of which experiences or mental representations are evoked through the realization of a mapping or conceptual projection—stored in our long-term memory or created as on-line representations (blends).

However, in the canonical western tradition, poetry follows a canon in relation to the classic idea of figurativeness and now also to the modern canons. Poets find their creative grounds in a comprehension (or a creative incomprehension) of the elements that create those conventions. According to Schmidt (1989: 16) we reach them coactivating:

1. a sense of tradition, given by allusion, interaction, influence or rhythm inside a tradition.
2. your senses given up to reading by means of analytic skills.
3. human voice which is the first and more incisive critical instrument and that even deceives both comprehension and incomprehension.

That implies the activation of our encyclopedic knowledge; the activation of basic metaphoric-conceptual knowledge (in our long-term memory) and integrative conceptual knowledge (in our active memory or working memory) which are fundamental cognitive means that affect any action or human thought (Turner and Fauconnier, 1995, 1997; Fauconnier and Turner, 1996, 2002; Grady, Okley and Coulson, 1999). These also activate interconnection between the semantic areas and those areas tightly related to sensorial perception or "receptor input" (visual, auditory, tactile, or bodily movements concepts) (Rohrer, 2002) and, lastly, the obtention of evoked meaning via condensation. The objective is to explain the "intuition" (Tsur, 1992: 250) through which the reader, or interpreter, perceives certain quality in a poem, and in that process of condensation encyclopedic knowledge has a great role with the activation of sense-relational nets or network activation (Graesser et al., 1997).

Cognitive schemas play an important role in this process of network activation. They are mental frameworks or structures that help us organize and process information metaphorically, including our perceptions, thoughts, and experiences (Lakoff and Johnson, 1999; Grady, 2005). These schemas play a crucial role in how we understand and make sense of the world around us. One specific type of cognitive schema is the trajector-landmark schema, which is often used to conceptualize spatial relationships and is associated with a specific cognitive linguist, Ronald Langacker (1987). Here's a brief overview of the trajector-landmark schema and a few other cognitive schemas:

1. TRAJECTOR-LANDMARK SCHEMA: This schema is a cognitive structure used to represent spatial relationships. It involves two key elements: Trajector, that is, the main object or entity whose spatial location or motion is being described, and Landmark, that is, the reference point or object with respect to which the trajector's location or motion is described. This schema helps us understand spatial prepositions like "in," "on," "under," and "between" by conceptualizing the relationships between objects or entities in space.
2. CONTAINER SCHEMA: The container schema is a cognitive structure used to understand containment relationships. It involves a container (an enclosing entity) and a contained entity. This schema is applied to various contexts, such as physical containment (e.g., a cup containing liquid) and abstract containment (e.g., a group containing members).
3. PATH SCHEMA: The path schema is used to conceptualize motion or movement along a path. It involves a moving entity (the trajector) and a path along which the entity moves. This schema helps us understand expressions like "go," "come," and "move" by organizing the motion conceptually.

4. SOURCE-GOAL SCHEMA: The source-goal schema represents a relationship between a source location and a goal location. It is often used to understand motion from one place to another. The source is where the motion originates, and the goal is the destination.
5. EVENT STRUCTURE SCHEMA: The event structure schema is a cognitive structure used to represent dynamic events. It involves components such as the participants (agents and patients), the action or process, and the result. This schema helps us conceptualize and understand events and actions in narratives and descriptions.
6. PART-WHOLE SCHEMA: The part-whole schema is used to represent relationships between a larger entity (whole) and its components or constituent parts. This schema helps us understand concepts of inclusion, hierarchy, and composition.

These cognitive schemas provide insights into how our minds structure and process various types of information, including spatial relationships, events, and conceptual categories.

The list of basic cognitive schemas continues to expand, encompassing concepts such as PENETRATION (Talmy, 2003: 216) and introducing others like the *BALANCE SCHEMA* (Johnson, 1987) and the *FAN SCHEMA* (Cortés de los Ríos and Bretones, 2016: 171). These schemas, rooted in our cognitive processes, provide insights into how our minds structure and interpret the world around us. The human mind is naturally attuned to the concept of balance and equilibrium. We have an intuitive understanding of balance, both physically (e.g., balancing objects) and metaphorically (e.g., balancing conflicting ideas). This intuitive sense of balance influences how we perceive and conceptualize various scenarios and can be easily represented in our mind. Spatial schemas like the trajector-landmark schema can play a role in understanding balance, especially when it involves physical objects. People often rely on spatial configurations to assess and maintain balance, whether it is arranging objects on a surface or distributing weight evenly. There are several logical possibilities for explaining the mental representations of fundamental units of experience, all of them connected to sensory experience.

As just mentioned above a spatial schema of balance can involve a trajectory-landmark structure in the understanding of something. People rely on their cognitive abilities to perceive and categorize patterns, whether they are geometric shapes or more abstract visual arrangements. Cognitive processes related to spatial organization, pattern recognition, and categorization (in the sense given by Rosch, 1978) are likely involved in understanding and interpreting fan-shaped displays as well. The concept of a "fan" refers to an object or device with a shape that resembles an open, spread-out hand-held fan, often used for cooling or decoration. The brain's pattern recognition mechanisms identify the fan's characteristic shape, which consists of multiple thin sections fanning out from a central point. Depending on the specific design of the fan, it may exhibit either radial symmetry (equal sections radiating from a central point) or asymmetry (sections differ in size, shape, or orientation). Symmetry tends to be aesthetically pleasing and easier to process, while asymmetry may draw attention and evoke different cognitive responses.

Cultural factors can influence how fans are perceived and interpreted. In some cultures, fans hold specific symbolic meanings or associations (e.g., as fashion accessories, status symbols or cultural artifacts). Contextual factors, such as where the fan is displayed or how it is used, can also impact perception. The fan shape can be mentally represented and processed as a category or prototype (cf. Rosch, 1978). People categorize objects based on shared features, and the fan's shape is often categorized as a subset of shapes that fan out or radiate from a central point. A fan-shaped display may attract visual attention due to its distinctive shape and arrangement. The contrast between the central point and the fanning sections can create a salient focal point that draws viewers' gaze (Cortés de los Ríos and Bretones, 2016). The concept of a fan can be metaphorically extended to describe other phenomena. For example, "fan out" can metaphorically refer to the spreading or dispersal of information, people, or objects from a central source. Overall, the perception and conception of a fan or a fan-shaped display involve a combination of perceptual mechanisms, cognitive processes, cultural influences, and context. These factors contribute to how individuals recognize, categorize, and interpret the visual pattern presented by the fan's distinct shape.

The schemas of balance and fan can be found in Heaney's poems. In the poem "Digging," Heaney portrays the balance between generations, acknowledging his roots in a family of laborers while embracing his role as a poet. The act of digging itself can be seen as a form of balance between tradition and progress. This balance is further nuanced by the spreading of the poem's imagery, similar to the fanning out concept, as Heaney connects his family's digging history to his own creative pursuit.

The fan schema, with its characteristic shape radiating from a central point, can be discerned in Heaney's poems. While not explicitly about fans, Heaney's poetry often captures the essence of spreading or radiating concepts. The fan as schematic conceptual structure represented metaphorically to provide the understanding of spreading and never being detached from its departure point. It is different from the source-goal schema because there is a sense of belonging to and coming back to the source that other schemas like the one just mentioned lack. In the poem "The Underground" (Station Island 1984) Heaney depicts the spreading roots of a tree that invoke the image of fanning out. This visual metaphor connects the natural world to the idea of growth and expansion, reflecting the concept of fanning out as seen in the fan schema. The image evokes the sense of reaching out from a central point, suggesting a metaphorical balance between grounded roots and expansive growth. He might use the metaphor of fanning out to depict the way a river's tributaries spread out from its source, or the way tree branches reach outward from their trunk. This imagery captures the idea of expansion and growth, which can also symbolize the dissemination of meaning or emotion. In the context of this book, we might use an example of the metaphor of "fanning out" to describe the way a story, theme, or concept unfolds within the poem itself. This could be the progression of ideas in the poem, where they start from a central point and then expand into a fuller exploration. It could also be used to describe the way emotions intensify and radiate through the lines of the poem.

Heaney represents this schema in poems such as "The Oak-Tree," where the tree symbolizes the stability and continuity of the natural world in contrast to the transient human existence: "Live oak, dead oak,/Oak within oak, looped around by osier/And groping up at daylight: as for the roots/You can use your hand to trace them." "Bogland" is another poems that while not explicitly about roots or trees, shows the bog, with its layers of peat, is a symbolic representation of the deep roots of Irish history and culture: "Our pioneers keep striking/Inwards and downwards,/Every layer they strip/Seems camped on before."

As we have just seen, Heaney often uses natural elements like roots, trees, and the land to explore themes of heritage, identity, and continuity. These examples show how skillfully he makes them symbols, and how the mental schema that allows us to grasp them is the fan schema structuring a sense of spreading but never departing from the origin, its departing point. This is the way in which cognitive structures enrich our experience and understanding, offering layers of meaning, emotional depth, and intellectual engagement.

4.2 Story, Cognitive Involvement and Affective Involvement

Cognitive involvement and affective involvement are two important factors that can influence the understanding and interpretation of a short story (Brosch, 2014; Toolan, 2012: 224). Cognitive involvement refers to a reader's concern with the functional information content of a communication, such as the plot, characters, and themes of a story (Brosch, 2014). In the context of a short story, cognitive involvement can influence how a reader processes and comprehends the narrative, including their ability to understand the sequence of events, identify the key themes and motifs, and interpret the actions and motivations of the characters. Affective involvement, on the other hand, refers to a reader's concern with the emotional and value-expressive content of a communication, such as the mood, tone, and symbolic significance of a story. In the context of a short story, affective involvement can influence how a reader responds to the narrative on an emotional level, including their ability to empathize with the characters, appreciate the aesthetic qualities of the language and imagery, and connect with the underlying themes and messages of the story.

Both cognitive and affective involvement are important for a reader to fully engage with and understand a short story. A reader who is highly cognitively involved may be able to follow the narrative and identify the key themes and motifs of a story but may miss the emotional nuances and symbolic significance that add depth and richness to the narrative. Conversely, a reader who is highly affectively involved may be able to appreciate the aesthetic and emotional qualities of the story but may struggle to fully comprehend the underlying themes and meanings. However, readers of short stories compress semantic units in a "synchronic reflective act" which encodes meaning "iconically" in a memorable way,—Brown refers to these iconic compressions as "configurations" (Brown, 1989: 242–243). These condensed images or parts of images have an intensifying effect that encourages projection and enhances memorability (Herman, 2002: 85).

In "Requiem for the Croppies," for example, Heaney (1966) uses language and symbolism to convey a sense of loss and mourning for the victims of the war:

> The pockets of our greatcoats full of barley—
> No kitchens on the run, no striking camp—
> We moved quick and sudden in our own country.
> The priest lay behind ditches with the tramp.
> A people hardly marching—on the hike—
> We found new tactics happening each day:
> We'd cut through reins and rider with the pike
> And stampede cattle into infantry,
> Then retreat through hedges where cavalry must be thrown.

Through this use of language and symbolism, Heaney is able to create an emotional connection with the reader, helping them to empathize with the victims of the war and to understand the human toll of political conflict.

Cognitive and affective involvement are two important factors that can affect a reader's understanding and interpretation of a short story (Stansfield and Bunce, 2014). A balance between these two forms of involvement can help a reader to fully engage with the narrative, appreciate its aesthetic and emotional qualities, and understand its underlying themes and meanings. They are both important factors in the interpretation of Seamus Heaney's poems about the Spanish Civil War. Through his use of vivid imagery and descriptive language, Heaney is able to convey the historical context and significance of the events he is describing, while through his use of language and symbolism, he is able to create an emotional connection with the reader, helping them to empathize with the victims of the war and to understand its human toll.

From a Cognitive Linguistics perspective, affective involvement refers to the emotional engagement, resonance, and subjective experience that individuals have with language and linguistic expressions. It acknowledges that language is not only a tool for communication but also a means to evoke and convey emotions, feelings, and affective states. Affective involvement recognizes that our understanding of language and the meaning we derive from it are deeply intertwined with our emotional responses. As seen in the previous one, Seamus Heaney's poems often exemplify affective involvement through the evocative language he uses to connect with readers on an emotional level. Here are some lines from Heaney's poems that demonstrate affective involvement:

1. From "Blackberry-Picking": "Each year I hoped they'd keep, knew they would not." These lines evoke a sense of fleetingness and disappointment, tapping into the reader's emotions of anticipation and eventual letdown.
2. From "Mid-Term Break": "A four-foot box, a foot for every year." These lines convey the stark reality of death and loss, eliciting feelings of sadness and empathy from the reader.
3. From "Digging": "Between my finger and my thumb The squat pen rests; snug as a gun." These lines create a vivid sensory image that appeals to touch and visual perception, while also hinting at deeper themes, triggering both sensory and emotional responses.
4. From "Clearances": "And they're waiting for me now—Those ones who had all the answers." These lines capture a sense of longing and nostalgia, as the speaker reflects on memories of loved ones who have passed away.
5. From "The Forge": "All I know is a door into the dark." This line resonates with a sense of uncertainty and exploration, inviting readers to reflect on their own journeys and experiences.

In each of these examples, Heaney's language evokes emotions, creating affective involvement by allowing readers to connect with the themes, imagery, and experiences depicted in the poems. The cognitive linguistic perspective recognizes that our emotional responses to language are inseparable from our cognitive processing, highlighting the intricate interplay between language, emotion, and cognition in the way we engage with texts.

Other examples of affective involvement can be found in the poems that will be analyzed in depth in Chapter 4:

1. "The First Words": "My only drink is meaning from the deep brain, What the birds and the grass and the stones drink." These lines evoke a sense of introspection and connection with nature, engaging the reader's emotions by portraying a unique perspective on the speaker's experience of "meaning" and its connection to the natural world.
2. "Remembered Columns": "Rose like remembered columns in a story About the Virgin's house that rose and flew And landed on the hilltop at Loreto." These lines evoke a feeling of reverence and nostalgia, inviting the reader to emotionally engage with the imagery of columns and the spiritual significance of the Virgin's house in Loreto.
3. "Lint Water": "Putrid currents floated trout to the loch, Their bellies white as linen tablecloths." These lines elicit a visceral reaction by describing the contaminated water's impact on the trout, conveying a sense of unease and environmental concern that can resonate with the reader's emotions.
4. "Sruth": "You in your dishabills Washing your face In the guttural glen." These lines evoke a sense of intimacy and vulnerability, allowing the reader to emotionally connect with the speaker's vivid memory of a person in a simple, unguarded moment.

In each of these examples, Heaney's use of imagery, language, and themes generates affective involvement by tapping into the reader's emotions, drawing them into the experiences and situations depicted in the poems. This demonstrates Heaney's ability to create a powerful emotional connection with his readers, a hallmark of his skill as a poet.

4.3 Voice, Technique and Synesthetic Metaphors in Heaney

Voice and technique are important for Seamus Heaney and they can both be conceived thanks to the metaphoric connections provided by his synesthetic force. According to Heaney (1980: 43) "finding a voice means that you can get your own feelings into your own words and that your words have the feel of you about them." Metaphor represents a way of handling the relative inability of language to account for, or directly express, the complexity of feeling. Heaney describes his own experience by saying that words have a particular way of feeling associated to each of them and how each person articulates them.

What one feels is not so easily transmitted and the ability to reason explicitly requires the logical manipulation of imagery (Damasio, 2021: 42). As Cacciari (1998: 127) noted, linguistic metaphors are verbal devices based on a sensory logic at the semantic level, and this entails a movement from abstract to concrete. It also involves the introduction of affect and the notion of perceptual qualities. Metaphor, with its capacity to introduce a sensory logic at the semantic level, is a way to fill this gap, for overcoming the rigidity of plain, straight, meaning and experiences of the world.

Technique, another of Heaney's preoccupations (1980: 47), can be defined as:

> the discovery of ways to go out of his normal cognitive bounds and ride the inarticulate: a dynamic alertness that mediates between the origins of feeling in memory and experience and the formal ploys that express this in a work of art. Technique entails the watermarking of your essential patterns of perception, voice and thought into the touch and texture of your lines; it is that whole creative effort of the mind's and body's resources to bring the meaning of experience within the jurisdiction of form.

Metaphor is based on experiential, body-linked, physical core of reasoning abilities. Metaphor has the capacity to introduce a sensory logic at the semantic level alluding to a more complex scenario of interrelated meanings and experiences of the world (Cacciari, 1998: 128). One of the most common types of metaphoric transfer is synesthesia (Williams, 1976: 463), that is, the transfer of information from one sensory modality to another. We can see some examples at work below (1–3):

1). The cold smell of potato mould, the squelch and slap
Of soggy peat, the curt cuts of an edge
Through living roots awaken in my head.
(Digging, lines 25–27);
SMELL IS TEMPERATURE
SMELLING IS FEELING

2). Yet I live here, I live here too, I sing,
Expertly civil-tongued with civil neighbours
On the high wires of first wireless reports,
Sucking the fake taste, the stony flavours
Of those sanctioned, old, elaborate retorts:
(From Whatever You Say Say Nothing, lines 16–20);
A FLAVOUR IS A STONY OBJECT
TASTING IS TOUCHING

3). Then one hot day when fields were rank
With cowdung in the grass the angry frogs
Invaded the flax-dam; I ducked through hedges
To a coarse croaking that I had not heard
Before. The air was thick with a bass chorus.
(Death of a Naturalist, lines 23–26);
SOUND QUALITY IS PHYSICAL TEXTURE
HEARING IS TOUCHING

Following this, in a corpus of fifty poems chosen randomly from Heaney's poems written before 1996, thirty-three cases of synesthetic metaphors were identified and the most prominent conceptual metaphors found were:

HEARING IS SEEING (21%)
HEARING IS TOUCHING (21%)
SEEING IS TOUCHING (12%)
TASTING IS TOUCHING (6%)
HEARING IS TASTING (6%)
HEARING IS FEELING (6%)
SEEING IS HEARING (6%)
TOUCHING IS FEELING (3%)
SMELLING IS FEELING (3%)
HEARING IS SMELLING (3%)
FEELING IS SMELLING (3%)
TOUCHING IS SEEING (3%)

FEELING IS SEEING (3%)
TOUCHING IS TASTING (3%)

These metaphors could be considered primary metaphors (Grady, 1999; Bretones, 2001), since there is a clear experiential correlation as their motivation and since other metaphors develop from them or share their "main meaning focus" or "scope of metaphor,"—as Kövecses calls it (2000: 81). Each source domain highlights one or a limited number of aspects of a target. The scope of metaphor allows us to make maximal generalizations about the use of particular source domains, thus making it possible to discover new systems of metaphors as the one presented here.

With this information, we can propose a model of metaphoric transfer different from that established by Cacciari (1998: 129), and to argue against Ullman (1964) and Cacciari (1998) when they say that the correspondence between modalities follows from the structure more distinctive modality to less distinctive modality. What Ullman calls less differentiated senses would be smell and taste, the more differentiated hearing and seeing. The very nature of perception can be characterized by an accurate and reliable receptive manipulation of data. Some researches have suggested that vision is very important, more so than other senses. The sense of smell is not weaker than that of other perception domains like hearing or vision (Ibarretxe, 1999: 41). The connection between smell and memory is very strong. Heiz (cited in Ibarretxe, 1999: 37) has found that memories evoked by the sense of smell are more emotional than those evoked by other senses, including vision, hearing and touch.

As we have mentioned before, Cacciari (1998) affirms that the main transfers in metaphors are those of the ruling sensory transfers. The metaphors found in Heaney show different information. The sensory transfer takes places from any sensory modality whenever we map conceptual structure from the source to the target domain. We could make extended comparisons between our data and the results showed by Cacciari (1999), but the general conclusions can be seen in the diagrams in Figures 5 and 6.

The present analysis reflects a model of metaphorical transfer between the sensory modalities different from the one given by Cacciari. In Heaney, Cacciari's order does not make sense; but the following diagram shows what Heaney is actually doing.

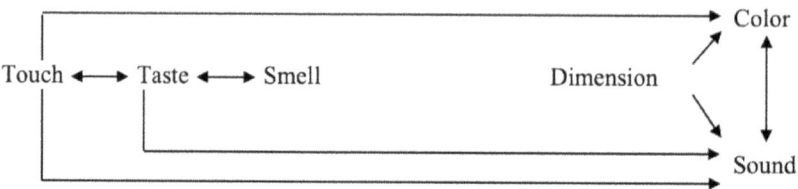

Figure 5. General model of metaphorical transfers among sensory modalities (Cacciari, 1998: 129, after Williams, 1976).

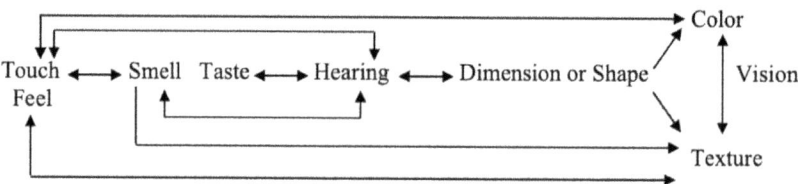

Figure 6. Model of metaphorical transfers among sensory modalities in the poetry of Seamus Heaney (Bretones, 2001).

1. Touch is mapped onto (see Figure 5):
   - taste, like in "sharp taste" (TASTING IS TOUCHING, 6%)
   - color, like in "dull color" (in our analysis we attribute color to the domain of seeing SEEING IS TOUCHING, 12%)
   - or sound, like in "soft sound" (HEARING IS TOUCHING-21%; HEARING IS FEELING, 6%).

According to Cacciari there are rare shifts to vision or smell, but our data shows the opposite. We find (see Figure 6):

   - vision, like in "milky gleam"[1] (SEEING IS TOUCHING, 21%)
   - smell, like in "cold smell" (SMELLING IS FEELING, 3%)
   - touch, like in "cold hardness" (TOUCHING IS FEELING, 3%)

[1] A gleam is defined as a pale, clear light (Collins Cobuild Dictionary), a steady bright shine, or a beam of light, often reflected, dim, or coming from an indistinct source (Encarta). Thus, the adjective 'milky' suggests something beyond mere whiteness in the light, as light itself inherently conveys a sense of illumination unless specified otherwise.

2. Taste is mapped onto:
   - Smell, like in "sour smell" (SMELLING IS TASTING, 0%)
   - and hearing, like in "sweet music" (HEARING IS TASTING, 6%).

But according to Cacciary smell does not map onto:

   - touch ("sweet hold," TOUCHING IS TASTING, 3%) or dimension (SHAPE IS TASTING, 0%) or color (COLOR IS TASTING, 0%). We find backward direction in Heaney,—towards touch.
3. Smell is not mapped onto any other sense according to Cacciari, but it is according to our data ("gauze of sound around the noise," HEARING IS SMELLING, 3%; "inhale the absolute weather," FEELING IS SMELLING, 3%).
4. Dimension is mapped onto
   - color, "flat grey"
   - or sound, "deep sound."

Cacciari mentions dimension without specifying texture or form. We did look for COLOR IS DIMENSION specifically or any other metaphor that identifies that quality in objects such as form, dimension and texture because we considered those included in vision or touch. The same happens with temperature, omitted by Cacciari (1998) and considered here as feeling.

5. Hearing is transferred only to color ("quiet green" COLOR IS HEARING, 0%). This statement made by Cacciari is not right according to my data. We find hearing transferred to another sensory modality, vision, like in "Smoke-signals are loud-mouthed" SEEING IS HEARING, 6%. But not to color.

The problem of directionality in synesthetic language has been mentioned by authors such as Ullman or Cacciari (1999). They show that the correspondence between senses is normally the one from the most distinctive modality (sight) to the lessen one (touch). But analysis presented here suggests strongly that this is not the case. It is true that there is a systematic directionality in the mapping, but not showing that the meaning that the metaphor conveys is presented by a term that belongs to the highest in the scale of distinction, while the modifying term belongs to the lowest modality in the scale. It is true that a mapping from more accessible or basic concepts seems more natural, and is preferred to its opposite, as shown by Shen (1997: 51), but that accessibility will function according to the meaning intended or perceived, never according to more or less accessible sensory modalities.

The proportion of metaphors in Heaney having vision as primary sense is much higher than the average one. "Seeing" is higher than "hearing" as primary sense too and touch has also much more significance in Heaney (Figure 6). Regarding the synesthetic use of the senses we must point out the fact that Heaney uses more touch, and in second place seeing (thought the difference is small). Taste and smell are the senses less used by Heaney in both groups.

All in all, Heaney's voice, as he describes, involves encapsulating his own feelings into words that authentically reflect his identity, creating a tangible sense of the poet's presence within the text. This personal infusion into language is crucial, as metaphor serves as a fundamental tool for expressing the inexpressible, bridging the gap between complex emotions and the constraints of language. The use of synesthetic metaphors, where sensory experiences are interchanged (like describing sounds in terms of colors or tastes in terms of touch), plays a fundamental role in Heaney's poetry. These metaphors not only enrich the semantic texture of his work but also enable a deeper sensory and emotional engagement with the reader. By transmuting the abstract into the concrete through these sensory crossovers, Heaney creates a more visceral, palpable poetic experience that mirrors the complexity of human perception and emotion. His poetry shows a dynamic range of sensory transfers, with a particularly notable use of touch, thereby providing a robust sensory foundation for his metaphoric structures. This synesthetic technique not only highlights his distinctive voice but also embodies his poetic technique, making the abstract palpable and the palpable profound.

CHAPTER 5

Textual Analysis

5.1 Integrated Textual Analysis Model

The method of textual analysis presented in this chapter offers a structured approach for thoroughly understanding and interpreting texts. This methodology aligns with the overarching framework outlined in Chapter 2, section 2.2, known as the Cognitive Linguistics Approach. It encompasses several essential components, each focused on different facets of the text to reveal its deeper meaning, metaphorical elements, synesthetic potential, cognitive blending, emotional impact, contextual backdrop, reader's view, and thematic exploration.

At the forefront is the identification of metaphors within the text. Metaphors involve attributing properties of one concept to another, creating layers of meaning. The analysis involves unraveling how these metaphors contribute to the text's overarching message or theme. Then, the exploration of Synesthetic potential follows, seeking elements that evoke sensory experiences across different senses. While the text might not overtly describe synesthetic encounters, it might contain word combinations prompting readers to imagine sensorial connections. A third step analyzes Cognitive blending, the process of merging distinct cognitive domains to create new meanings, is then examined. This uncovers how the text weaves together various concepts or ideas, enhancing its complexity and offering deeper insights. Emotional resonance is another critical consideration, focusing on the impact of the text on readers' emotions. The analysis shows how metaphors, synesthetic elements, and cognitive blends contribute to the text's emotional depth and influence on readers' feelings and reactions. Contextual analysis becomes fundamental to situate the text within its broader context. This involves considering the author's background, historical setting, literary genre, and other influences that add layers of significance to the text (Guerra, 2019; Pereira, 2019). Finally, interpreting the text through the reader's perspective is also integral. This involves examining how metaphors, synesthetic elements, cognitive blends, and emotional resonances shape readers' understanding and engagement. And last, but not least, thematic exploration entails investigating the central themes or ideas conveyed by the text. Reflecting on how metaphors, synesthetic potential, cognitive blending, and emotional resonances contribute to these themes enriches the interpretation.

By employing this analytical model, a systematic study of a text's dimensions unfolds (Figure 7). This approach uncovers nuanced metaphors, sensory evocations, cognitive intricacies, emotional impacts, and more, ultimately enriching the interpretation and appreciation of the author's craftsmanship. For a more detailed description, each step of the model could be expanded as follows, offering a comprehensive framework that shows multiple layers of meaning, engages with sensory and emotional dimensions, and connects the text to its context and readers' experiences.

Here's a comprehensive overview:

1. Metaphoric Potential:
   - Explore the origins and cultural connotations of specific metaphors in the text.
   - Analyze how metaphors evolve or transform throughout the text, revealing shifts in meaning.
   - Consider the potential interplay between different metaphors within the text and how they contribute to its complexity.
2. Synesthetic Potential:
   - Go deeper into the sensory associations evoked by specific phrases or words.
   - Investigate how synesthetic potential varies across different sections of the text and its impact on pacing and tone.
   - Examine whether synesthetic elements connect to specific characters, themes, or narrative arcs.
3. Cognitive Blending:
   - Explore how cognitive blending can create layers of meaning that resonate with different audiences.

Textual Analysis

- Consider how cognitive blending reflects the text's themes and contributes to its overall structure.
- Analyze how blending might involve concepts from various cultural, historical, or artistic domains.

4. Emotional Resonance:
   - Evaluate the potential for ambivalence or conflicting emotions generated by metaphors, synesthetic elements, and blending.
   - Examine the relationship between emotional resonance and the text's pacing, characterization, and plot development.
   - Reflect on how emotional resonances may differ based on readers' backgrounds and perspectives.
5. Contextual Analysis:
   - Investigate the social, political, or philosophical context of the text's creation and consider how it influences the themes and metaphors.
   - Explore how the text engages with literary traditions or responds to other works within its genre.
   - Examine the impact of the author's personal experiences on the text's content and style.
6. Reader's Perspective:
   - Consider the influence of reader expectations, cultural backgrounds, and personal experiences on interpretation.
   - Reflect on the potential for diverse readings and how multiple interpretations contribute to the richness of the text.
   - Explore the text's potential for engaging readers emotionally, intellectually, and philosophically.
7. Thematic Exploration:
   - Analyze how metaphors, synesthetic potential, cognitive blending, and emotional resonances contribute to the exploration of specific themes.
   - Investigate how these elements evolve or shift as the text progresses, reflecting changes in narrative focus.
   - Consider how the interplay of various elements contributes to the text's overarching message or commentary.

Expanding the model in these comprehensive ways holds the potential to facilitate more profound analyzes, enabling the revelation of layers of meaning that might otherwise remain concealed. By approaching the text from various angles, we embark on a journey that unveils additional dimensions, enriching our interpretation. However, it is essential to bear in mind that while these expansions offer a broader framework, flexibility remains paramount. We shall adeptly tailor the model to align with the distinctive qualities inherent in each text under analysis. This dynamic adaptation ensures that our approach remains attuned to the intricacies of the text while adhering to a structured methodology that elevates our comprehension and appreciation of literature.

Least, but not least, within this extended framework, it is important to considering the conceptualization of storytelling, with its (1) beginning, its (2) middle and its (3) end. It can be viewed as a condensed narrative that conveys a thematic message, leading to its "iconic power." Iconic power, referring to the ability of language and imagery to create lasting impressions on the reader, introduces a layer of meaning that can be explored. Uncovering instances of iconic power within the text adds depth to our analysis, unveiling how the author harnesses linguistic elements to evoke vivid mental imagery and sensory experiences, thereby intensifying the reader's engagement.

Moreover, the cultural context provided by the text adds a critical dimension. Literature is often intertwined with cultural nuances, and by examining how the text resonates with cultural elements, symbols, or traditions, we gain insights into how it connects with broader societal narratives and values. This exploration enhances our understanding of the text's significance within its cultural milieu. Affective involvement, too, emerges as a crucial consideration. As we traverse the text's emotional resonances, we see the ways in which the author's use of metaphors, synesthetic elements, and cognitive blends triggers emotional responses in the reader. By dissecting the interplay between language and emotion, we discern how the text forges a profound emotional connection, fostering a lasting impact.

Analytical Framework	Key Aspects	Focus Areas
1. Metaphoric Potential	- Explore origins and connotations of metaphors	- Evolution/Transformation of metaphors - Interplay between metaphors - Contribution to text's complexity
2. Synesthetic Potential	- Pinpoint the sensory associations	- Variation across text sections - Impact on pacing and tone - Connection to characters, themes, or narrative arcs
3. Cognitive Blending	- Deepen layers of meaning through blending	- Reflection of themes - Contribution to text structure - Involvement of cultural, historical, or artistic concepts
4. Emotional Resonance	- Assess ambivalence or conflicting emotions	- Relationship with pacing, characterization, and plot - Variation based on reader background - Influence of metaphors, synesthetic elements, and blending
5. Contextual Analysis	- Analyze social, political, philosophical context	- Engagement with literary traditions - Response to other works in the genre - Influence of author's personal experiences
6. Reader's Perspective	- Consider influence of reader expectations	- Potential for diverse interpretations - Contribution to text richness - Emotional, intellectual, and philosophical engagement
7. Thematic Exploration	- Analyze contributions of metaphors, synesthesia, blending, emotional resonance	- Evolution of themes throughout the text - Shifts in narrative focus - Contribution to overarching message or commentary
8. Short Story Structure	- Focus on narrative structure (Beginning, Middle, End)	- Analysis of "iconic power" in language - Uncovering instances of vivid imagery and lasting impressions
9. Iconic Power	- Explore how language/imagery create lasting impressions	- Identification of vivid mental imagery - Examination of sensory experiences - Contribution to reader's engagement
10. Cultural Context	- Investigate connection with cultural elements, symbols, or traditions	- Insights into societal narratives and values - Enhancing understanding of text within its cultural milieu
11. Affective Involvement	- Dissect emotional connections through language	- Analysis of emotional triggers - Interplay between language and emotion - Examination of how text forges lasting emotional impact
Overall Approach	- Flexibility and dynamic adaptation	- Tailoring the model to text's distinctive qualities - Ensuring comprehensive analysis while remaining structured and flexible to explore textual intricacies and cultural implications

Figure 7. Integrated Textual Analysis Model (ITAM)

In sum, by integrating the elements of short story, iconic power, cultural context, and affective involvement into the expanded model, we provide a comprehensive analytical approach that addresses the multifaceted nature of literature. This enriched methodology allows us to engage with the text on multiple levels, uncovering its inherent complexities, cultural implications, and emotional resonances. Flexibility remains our guiding principle, enabling us to adapt and tailor the model while adhering to its structured framework, thereby enhancing our explorations of the textual subtleties.

The following sections explore various applications of the model of analysis developed here, the ITAM, highlighting its flexibility and effectiveness in uncovering subtle textual meanings.

5.2 The Haw Lantern

Seamus Heaney's poem "The Haw Lantern," published in his 1987 poetry collection of the same name and renowned for its exploration of themes such as personal integrity, moral scrutiny, and the resilience of the human spirit, shall serve as an exemplar for the model of analysis displayed in previous section and, as already mentioned in this book—more specifically when referring to the subject of poetry (Hughes, 1993: 47)—, of Heaney's capacity to provide through his poems a story as an exemplar to teach or explain. Here is the poem and its analysis following the ITAM:

> The wintry haw is burning out of season,
> crab of the thorn, a small light for small people,
> wanting no more from them but that they keep
> the wick of self-respect from dying out,
> not having to blind them with illumination.
>
> But sometimes when your breath plumes in the frost
> it takes the roaming shape of Diogenes
> with his lantern, seeking one just man;
> so you end up scrutinized from behind the haw
> he holds up at eye-level on its twig,

and you flinch before its bonded pith and stone,
its blood-prick that you wish would test and clear you,
its pecked-at ripeness that scans you, then moves on.

1. Metaphoric Potential
   – The "haw lantern" itself is a central metaphor, symbolizing a small but significant source of light or hope during difficult times.
   – The "wintry haw" burning "out of season" suggests resilience and survival despite adverse conditions.
   – The metaphor evolves from a simple representation of a hawthorn berry to a deeper symbol of self-respect and moral integrity.
   – The reference to Diogenes, the ancient Greek philosopher known for his quest for an honest man, adds layers of philosophical inquiry to the metaphor. The small, resilient light of the haw lantern contrasts with the grander but often blinding illumination of greater truths or moral judgments.
2. Synesthetic Potential
   – The imagery of the hawthorn berry as a "small light" invokes both visual and tactile sensations. Readers can picture the glowing red of the berry and feel its small, round shape.
   – The phrase "your breath plumes in the frost" evokes a sensory blend of sight (the visible breath in cold air) and touch (the chill of the frost).
   – These sensory details contribute to a contemplative and introspective tone, encouraging readers to reflect on the subtle sources of light and hope in their own lives.
   – The synesthetic imagery connects to the themes of endurance, moral scrutiny, and the search for authenticity.
3. Cognitive Blending
   – The poem blends the natural image of the hawthorn with the philosophical quest of Diogenes, creating a rich picture that bridges the natural and intellectual realms.
   – The concept of a lantern held by Diogenes searching for an honest man merges with the hawthorn berry's small light, symbolizing an ongoing quest for integrity and truth.

- This blend reinforces the poem's themes of moral scrutiny, the search for truth, and the resilience of the human spirit. It draws from historical and philosophical domains, particularly Greek philosophy and Celtic mythology, enriching the poem's resonance.
4. Emotional Resonance
    - The poem evokes a mixture of hope and discomfort. The haw lantern's light symbolizes hope, yet the scrutiny it represents can be unsettling.
    - The poem's steady pacing and contemplative tone support its emotional resonance, allowing readers to dwell on the imagery and its implications.
    - Readers may experience varying emotional responses based on their own experiences with moral scrutiny and the quest for integrity.
5. Contextual Analysis
    - Written in the context of Heaney's reflections on personal and societal integrity, the poem could be seen as a response to the moral and political challenges of his time, including the Troubles in Northern Ireland.
    - The poem engages with the tradition of philosophical poetry, drawing on classical references and Irish mythological elements to deepen its themes.
    - Heaney's own experiences growing up in a politically turbulent environment influence the poem's exploration of moral scrutiny and the search for personal integrity.
6. Reader's Perspective
    - Readers familiar with Heaney's work may expect themes of nature and moral inquiry, which are indeed present in the poem.
    - The poem invites multiple interpretations, allowing readers to see it as a meditation on personal integrity, a commentary on societal morals, or a reflection on the natural world's resilience.
    - The poem engages readers both intellectually and emotionally, encouraging them to reflect on their own moral standing and the sources of light in their lives.

7. Thematic Exploration
   – The poem explores themes of moral scrutiny, the search for truth, and the endurance of hope and integrity in difficult times. As the poem progresses, it moves from a simple depiction of a hawthorn berry to a deeper meditation on the nature of moral inquiry and personal integrity.

The interplay of metaphors, sensory imagery, and cognitive blends enhances the poem's overarching message, emphasizing the importance of maintaining self-respect and seeking truth. The haw lantern's image holds iconic power, symbolizing a small but resilient source of light and hope. The poem's cultural context, particularly Irish mythology and the historical backdrop of Northern Ireland, adds depth to its themes and metaphors. The poem's affective involvement is also very significant, evoking a range of emotions from hope to unease, mirroring the reader's own experiences with moral scrutiny and the quest for authenticity.

By applying this analytical model, we not only uncover the metaphors, sensory evocations, cognitive intricacies, and emotional impacts of "The Haw Lantern." This structured approach reveals the poem's rich layers of meaning, enhancing our interpretation and appreciation of Seamus Heaney's craftsmanship. The model's flexibility ensures that our analysis remains attuned to the text's complexities, offering a comprehensive framework that deepens our understanding of the poem. In addition, considering the conceptualization of storytelling with the beginning, middle, and end of the story can reveal a condensed narrative that conveys a thematic message. This storytelling structure and the poem's "iconic power"—the ability of its language and imagery to create lasting impressions—add layers of meaning and enhance reader engagement.

The poem shows the following storytelling structure:

- Beginning:

The poem opens with the image of "The wintry haw … burning out of season," immediately presenting a striking, vivid metaphor. This sets the stage for the poem, introducing the central symbol of the haw lantern, which represents a small but persistent light in the darkness. The mention of "small people" and "self-respect" establishes the theme of humble resilience.

- Middle:

The middle of the poem goes deeper into the symbolic and thematic elements, invoking the image of Diogenes with his lantern. Diogenes, a philosopher known for his search for an honest man, adds a layer of philosophical depth. The narrative unfolds as the speaker describes the haw lantern being used to scrutinize individuals, representing a quest for moral integrity. The breath forming into frost and taking the shape of Diogenes adds a dynamic and almost mystical quality to the narrative, enriching the theme of searching for truth and authenticity.

- End:

The poem concludes with the scrutiny of the haw lantern, which causes the subject to "flinch before its bonded pith and stone." This closing section brings the narrative to a poignant end, highlighting the discomfort and challenge of moral scrutiny. The final lines, "its blood-prick that you wish would test and clear you, its pecked-at ripeness that scans you, then moves on," emphasize the ongoing nature of this moral examination, leaving the reader with a lasting impression of the haw lantern's symbolic power.

The emotional impact of the poem is significant. The small, resilient light of the haw lantern serves as a metaphor for personal integrity and self-respect, evoking feelings of hope and admiration for those who maintain their moral compass despite difficult circumstances. At the same time, the scrutiny represented by the hawthorn's gaze can be unsettling, prompting readers to reflect on their own moral standing. By viewing "The Haw Lantern" as a condensed narrative with a clear beginning, middle, and end, we can appreciate the thematic message of resilience and moral scrutiny. The iconic power of the poem lies in its vivid language and imagery, which create lasting impressions and evoke sensory and emotional experiences.

This analysis uncovers the layers of meaning that Heaney displays in a poem, intensifying the reader's engagement and deepening our understanding. The following sections show further examples.

5.3 The First Words

Seamus Heaney's poem "The First Words," which is included in his poetry collection titled *The Spirit Level* (1996: 38), is one of Heaney's best collections and features poems that explore various themes, including politics, history, language, and the natural world. This is the poem "The First Words":

> The first words got polluted
> Like river water in the morning
> Flowing with the dirt
> Of blurb and the front pages.
> My only drink is meaning from the deep brain,
> What the birds and the grass and the stones drink.
> Let everything flow
> Up to the four elements,
> Up to water and earth and fire and air.

This poem specifically addresses the power and purity of language and its relationship with meaning and communication but let us use our model of textual analysis to see its intricacies. The structured approach presented in this chapter allows us to engage with the poem on multiple levels and appreciate the layers of meaning it conveys:

1. Metaphoric Potential:
   - The metaphor here is "river water in the morning" being compared to the "first words" that have become "polluted."
   - This metaphor suggests that the initial purity of "first words" has been tainted by external influences, like river waters becoming contaminated by impurities.
   - The metaphor conveys the idea of the deterioration of language and meaning due to the intrusion of superficial and commercial elements.
2. Synesthetic Potential:
   - The phrase "flowing with the dirt" has a synesthetic potential, evoking both visual and tactile imagery of dirt mixing with flowing water.

- This phrase invites readers to imagine the merging of two sensory experiences, enhancing the text's vividness and emotional resonance.
3. Cognitive Blending:
    - The phrase "My only drink is meaning from the deep brain" blends the concept of "drink" with "meaning," emphasizing the idea that the speaker seeks intellectual nourishment rather than literal refreshment.
    - The blending of "birds," "grass," and "stones" drinking emphasizes the interconnectedness of nature and the universality of seeking sustenance, whether physical or metaphorical.
4. Emotional Resonance:
    - The poem's imagery and metaphors evoke a sense of concern about the pollution of language and meaning by commercialism ("blurb and the front pages").
    - The idea of seeking "meaning from the deep brain" and the imagery of elements like "water and earth and fire and air" contribute to a contemplative tone, prompting readers to reflect on the essence of communication and knowledge.
5. Contextual Analysis:
    - The poem was written in 1995, a time when mass media and consumer culture were prevalent influences on language and communication.
    - Heaney's background as a renowned poet and his engagement with issues related to language, culture, and authenticity.
    - On August 31, 1994, the Provisional Irish Republican Army stunned the world by announcing a conditional ceasefire. This ceasefire did not last indefinitely: it was shattered in 1996 by devastating bombings in London and Manchester. Nevertheless, the Provisional IRA, once committed to absolute victory, now seemed willing to consider a negotiated peace.
6. Reader's Perspective:
    - Readers may connect with the theme of seeking genuine meaning amidst the noise of commercial language.

- Depending on readers' experiences, they might interpret the poem as a commentary on the degradation of language in the modern world.
7. Thematic Exploration:
    - The poem explores the idea of linguistic pollution and the search for genuine meaning within a society inundated with superficial language.
    - It also touches on the theme of interconnectedness, drawing parallels between human consumption of knowledge and the sustenance of nature.

The poem reflects on how words carry meaning and the power they hold, especially when they are the initial expressions that convey thoughts and ideas. In the poem, Heaney juxtaposes the purity of "first" with the potential pollution of language. He draws a parallel between the contamination of river water and the pollution of language through elements like commercialism and superficiality. This metaphor highlights the idea that language, like water, can be tainted by external influences, causing it to lose its original clarity and authenticity. The poem's focus on "meaning from the deep brain" suggests a longing for genuine, profound communication that goes beyond superficiality. This desire for meaningful connection resonates throughout the poem, as Heaney emphasizes the interconnectedness of all living things through the imagery of birds, grass, stones, and the elements.

When considering the conceptualization of storytelling in the context of this poem, we can view it as a condensed narrative that conveys a thematic message. While "The First Words" is a poem and not a traditional short story, it encapsulates a narrative essence through its progression of ideas and imagery.

The poem itself can be seen as a short story in miniature, with a clear beginning, middle, and end:

- Beginning: The introduction of "The first words got polluted," presenting the central concept of the poem.
- Middle: The comparison between contaminated river water and language's pollution through commercialism and superficiality.

- End: The speaker's reflection on seeking genuine meaning from the "deep brain" and the evocation of elements.

The thematic exploration of language, communication, and meaning creates a narrative arc within the poem. This narrative-like structure mirrors the condensed storytelling that can be found in short stories, where a compact form is used to convey a complete narrative arc and evoke emotions or insights.

In this way, "The First Words" can be appreciated as a brief narrative exploration within the realm of poetry, demonstrating how storytelling concepts can be encapsulated in even the most concise of literary forms.

From a cognitive perspective, when we read the poem, we select elements like "first" (line 1), "river water" (line 2), " morning" (line 2) and verbs like "pollute" or "flow" (line 2). We keep them in our short-term memory and play with them in search of general and integrated meaning. From our point of view, we are placed in a specific frame, that is, the one provided by the folk theory or the traditionally shared belief regarding to WHAT COMES FIRST IS PURE OR FIRST IS UNPOLLUTED. So that, "the first words," being "first" are "unpolluted," pristine, pure. "Morning" would also be related to it, because it would indicate the "first" hour of the day, when the atmosphere is cleaner and fresh air is breathed, and at that "first" hour the flowing water is pure and clean. In this way, we create our own relational structure in the elaboration of our networks of sense relation, activated in turn by what would be folk theory.

In this poem, our perception of the orientational relationship UP/DOWN is also activated. Through orientational primary metaphors (see Figure 4, and Lakoff and Johnson, 1999) such as MORE IS UP/LESS IS DOWN, which allow us to understand or structure terms in relation to others, we reach an understanding of the poem, since this directionality guides us in obtaining meaning. The positive quality is above and the negative below, the good above and the bad below, the pure above and the impure below, the free above and the forbidden below, the positive is above and the negative below. For example, we usually say "my morale is down" to express a bad emotional state, or lacking in positive qualities, or "your sympathy lifted my spirits," for the opposite. In the poem, elements such as "flow," associated with the idea of a liquid moving in a current and implicitly carrying an origin "up" but a direction "down," show a concrete tendency. It is a continuous going down, losing strength, losing purity, losing positive qualities. Other elements support this, such as "river," "water," "drink," "deep." But in line 8 there is an interruption of the "normal flow." We meet "up," with a concrete end represented by the metaphor PURPOSES ARE DESTINATIONS, indicating a beginning and a final destination in the journey of the "words."

The orientation INSIDE/OUT should not go unnoticed as well since it is reflected in the verb "drink" (line 5) and includes the metaphorical conception of the individual as a vessel with a limited surface and an inside and an outside. Limited objects, whether beings, rocks, or extensions of land, have size. That makes them susceptible to being quantified and measured or pigeonholed, and even "drunk" by our senses. In this same way, words, which have an exterior and a content, are quantified. Nature, culture, mind, brain, consciousness … affect words, affect language. It is in that flow, in that continuum (line 3 "flowing"), where we are affected, where words are contaminated, where we are (line 1) "polluted." But the purpose of that flowing of the mind we see in lines 8 and 9 when we come upon "up to." Here we are shown the DESTINATION of our flow, and it is none other than the four elements of nature, the origin and purity by essence (line 9), the most basic, as basic as a child's first words can be.

Understood in this way, we can see the poem as the story of a cycle, the cycle of water going from liquid to gaseous and back to liquid as it condenses again. It is the cyclical structure of the process of contamination and purification that permeates words, ideas, life.

5.4 Remembered Columns

This poem belongs to Seamus Heaney's collection titled "The Spirit Level" which was published in 1987. This collection, which features Heaney's reflective and contemplative poetry that often explores themes of memory, language, history, and the complexities of human experience. The poem "Remembered Columns" (1987: 45) reflects these qualities showing the transformation of language and imagery.

> The solid letters of the world grew airy.
> The marble serifs, the clearly blocked uprights
> Built upon rocks and set upon the heights
> Rose like remembered columns in a story
> About the Virgin's house that rose and flew
> And landed on the hilltop at Loreto.
> I lift my eyes in a light-headed credo,
> Discovering what survives translation true.

Following our model of textual analysis provided in Section 4.1, the following elements of the text might be highlighted:

1. Metaphoric Potential:
   - The phrase "The solid letters of the world grew airy" presents a metaphorical contrast between "solid letters" and "airy" ones.
   - The metaphor conveys a transformation of something concrete ("solid letters") into something ethereal or abstract ("airy"), suggesting a shift from physical to metaphorical or symbolic representation.
2. Synesthetic Potential:
   - The phrase "I lift my eyes in a light-headed credo" combines visual imagery ("lift my eyes") with the sensation of feeling "light-headed."
   - This blending creates a synesthetic experience by associating a visual action with a physical sensation, enhancing the reader's sensory engagement.
3. Cognitive Blending:
   - The line "Built upon rocks and set upon the heights" blends architectural imagery ("built upon rocks") with spatial imagery ("set upon the heights").
   - This blending merges concepts of construction and elevation, inviting readers to imagine the solidity of structures rising to elevated positions.

4. Emotional Resonance:
   - The poem's imagery of "remembered columns" and the reference to the "Virgin's house" evoke a sense of historical or religious significance.
   - The exploration of translation and what "survives translation true" adds an introspective layer, inviting contemplation about the enduring nature of meaning.
5. Contextual Analysis:
   - The reference to "The Virgin's house" and "Loreto" alludes to religious and cultural contexts, possibly referencing the Basilica della Santa Casa in Loreto, Italy.
   - The poem's exploration of translation could also reflect Heaney's interest in language, communication, and the challenges of conveying meaning across languages.
   - The most famous columns hit by the airy coasts of Norther Ireland are the ones that form the famous Giant's Causeway and evoke the famous legend of a giant called Finn McCool.
6. Reader's Perspective:
   - Readers may approach the poem with different levels of familiarity with religious and architectural references.
   - The contemplative tone and focus on translation could resonate with readers who have experienced the complexities of conveying meaning across languages or cultures.
7. Thematic Exploration:
   - The poem shows the transformation of the physical ("solid letters") into the abstract or ethereal ("airy").
   - Themes of preservation and transformation are explored through the metaphor of "remembered columns" and the discussion of translation.

In the poem, Heaney uses metaphors and vivid imagery to convey the transformation of solid letters into airy ones. The imagery of "remembered columns" and the reference to the Virgin's house landing at Loreto evoke a sense of historical and cultural significance. The poem also touches on the theme of translation and maybe the quest for meaning that transcends language barriers.

Some words are lexical keys to a general understanding of the text. Provided by its title, the word "Remembered" is an example. This word locates us in a specific frame, that is, at the frame of ideas and the metaphor IDEAS ARE A LOCATIONS activates. That general frame is a place where to read and integrate meaning from. That general frame is "the mind." The columns of the mind "grow airy" as they stand or elevate in an airy space and they are "clearly," that is, "easily, distinctly, lucidly or visually" accessible. We also find the expression "light-headed" implying feeling dizzy or not fully conscious until the discovery of "what survives translation true," that is, what makes ideas true and remains.

When considering the conceptualization of storytelling in the context of this poem, we can view it as a condensed narrative that conveys a thematic message. While the poem itself is not a traditional short story, it encapsulates a narrative essence through its progression of ideas and imagery. The poem's structure can be seen as a short story:

- Beginning: The introduction of the transformation of "solid letters" into "airy" ones.
- Middle: The description of "remembered columns" and the allusion to the Virgin's house at Loreto.
- End: The speaker's contemplative reflection on translation and the pursuit of enduring meaning.

This narrative-like structure within the poem mirrors the condensed storytelling often found in short stories. While the poem doesn't follow a linear plot, it encapsulates a thematic journey from concrete to abstract, invoking historical and spiritual dimensions along the way.

By seeing the poem as a form of condensed storytelling, readers can appreciate how Heaney's use of metaphors, imagery, and thematic exploration creates a narrative arc that invites reflection and contemplation, much like a short story does within a limited space.

5.5 Lint Water

The poem "Lint Water" was first published in *The Times Literary Supplement* on August 5, 1965. It was later included in Seamus Heaney's collection "Door into the Dark," which was first published in 1969. This collection is marked by Heaney's exploration of nature, rural life, and the complexities of human interaction with the environment. "Lint Water" is a powerful poem that vividly portrays the process of flax processing and its environmental consequences. The collection as a whole reflects Heaney's ability to use language and imagery to convey both the beauty and harsh realities of the natural world. One key aspect of interpreting the poem lies in understanding the term "lint," which the OED defines primarily as "(especially British English) a type of soft cotton cloth used for covering and protecting wounds." Secondary meanings include "(specialist) short fine fibers that come off the surface of cloth during its production" and "(especially North American English, in British English usually 'fluff') small soft pieces of wool, cotton, etc. that stick to the surface of cloth." In the context of the poem, however, "lint" may take on a metaphorical sense, suggesting dirt in the water. This is the poem:

> The flax was pulled by hand once it ripened,
> Bound into tall green pillars with rush bands
> And buried underwater, roots upwards.
> When the dam was full they loaded stones and sods
> On top, then left the whole thing for three weeks
> To rot, to stink: a pit of rotten eggs
> Could not have generated such a fug
> As flax decaying, steaming like a bog,
> Wafting its heavy, nauseating fall-out.
> As soon as stems had turned to slime and smut
> The dam was emptied: men stood waist deep
> In the fouled water, with fork and four-pronged grape
> Pitching out sheaves like half-gone carcasses.
> They spread it dripping, then, flat on the grass
> To crisp and dry hard in the summer sun
> Until it could be stooked up, stiff as broom
> And whistling in the wind. Toughened to sticks,

> The stems were milled, spun, woven into fabrics.
> The dam was cleared, poured down into the river
> Its poisonous bellyful. "Lint water"
> It was called. Across the stream it swirled brown froth
> That scummed clean stone and sickened fish to death;
> And if the drains were blocked, it still seeped down,
> Filtering unseen contamination.
> Putrid currents floated trout to the loch,
> Their bellies white as linen tablecloths.

Following our model of textual analysis, we might highlight the following elements from the text:

1. Metaphoric Potential:
   - The metaphor of "flax decaying, steaming like a bog" conveys the deterioration of the flax as a vivid and tangible image.
   - The description of the "poisonous bellyful" of the dam and the term "lint water" reflect the metaphorical aspect of language by attributing human-like qualities to natural elements.
2. Synesthetic Potential:
   - The phrase "wafting its heavy, nauseating fall-out" combines olfactory ("nauseating") and tactile ("heavy") sensations, creating a synesthetic experience that evokes a vivid sense of smell and weight.
3. Cognitive Blending:
   - The image of "men stood waist deep/In the fouled water, with fork and four-pronged grape/Pitching out sheaves like half-gone carcasses" blends agricultural imagery with a sense of decay and removal.
   - The term "lint water" blends two elements—"lint" and "water"—into a phrase that captures the essence of the process described in the poem.
4. Emotional Resonance:
   - The poem evokes emotions through visceral descriptions of decay and pollution, as well as the impact on the environment.

- The imagery of "poisonous bellyful" and "sickened fish to death" creates a sense of unease and concern for the consequences of human actions.
5. Contextual Analysis:
   - Published in 1965, this poem reflects Heaney's interest in rural life, labor, and the connection between humanity and the natural world.
   - It also echoes Heaney's exploration of the complexities and ambiguities of human relationships with nature and the environment.
6. Reader's Perspective:
   - Readers may respond emotionally to the poem's graphic descriptions, prompting reflection on environmental impact and human interaction with nature.
   - Different readers might bring personal experiences or cultural backgrounds that influence their interpretation.
7. Thematic Exploration:
   - The poem explores the process of harvesting and processing flax, but it also addresses pollution and environmental consequences.
   - Themes include the dual nature of human intervention in nature, the transformative power of human labor, and the unintended harm caused by industrial practices.

By applying the model of textual analysis, we can appreciate how Heaney employs metaphors, synesthetic potential, cognitive blending, emotional resonances, context, reader perspectives, and thematic exploration to create a multi-layered narrative that engages readers and prompts reflection on the complex relationships between humanity and the environment. In it he offers a vivid depiction of the process of harvesting and processing flax, along with the environmental consequences of these actions. The conflict in the poem is twofold—the struggle to process the flax while dealing with its pungent odor and the environmental consequences of polluting the dam and river. The poem addresses themes of human labor, environmental impact, and the consequences of industrial processes and this thematic exploration is similar to what short stories often convey through their narratives.

The poem embodies certain elements of storytelling and conceptualization within its condensed structure:

- Narrative Essence: The poem captures a narrative essence by presenting a series of events and actions that unfold in a sequential manner. It starts with the pulling of flax and progresses through its various stages until the final outcome.
- Setting and Characters: The poem's vivid descriptions provide a sense of setting—the flax fields, the dam, the river—while characters such as the workers engaged in the flax-processing activities are indirectly presented.
- Plot Progression: The poem follows a progression that resembles the arc of a short story, beginning with the initial harvesting, moving through the various stages of processing, and concluding with the impact on the environment.

In essence, while the poem is not a short story in its traditional sense, it encapsulates a narrative essence that follows a progression of events and explores themes and consequences. This condensed storytelling provides readers with a glimpse into a narrative structure that engages emotions and prompts reflection—characteristics shared with short stories. And, although the structure is more complex and fluid than a traditional narrative, the poem shows elements of a beginning, middle, and end.

- Beginning: The poem's beginning introduces the process of flax cultivation, describing how the flax is pulled by hand, bound into pillars, and submerged underwater. This initial section sets the stage for the subsequent events and themes of the poem.
- Middle: The middle section of the poem shows the consequences of submerging the flax underwater and leaving it to rot for three weeks. It vividly describes the foul odor and noxiousness that result from the decaying flax, using similes to evoke the sense of smell and imagery that portrays the degradation of the flax.
- End: The poem's end shifts focus to the aftermath of the flax's decay. It describes the process of emptying the dam, spreading the material

Textual Analysis 103

on grass to dry, and eventually processing it into fabrics. The final lines emphasize the contamination caused by pouring the "lint water" down the river, affecting the environment and its inhabitants.

While "Lint Water" doesn't follow a strict narrative arc, it does have a progression from the initial cultivation of flax to the consequences of its decay and the eventual processing of the material. The poem's structure reflects its thematic exploration of the industrial processes and environmental impact associated with flax cultivation. It draws attention to the delicate balance between human industry and the natural world. It portrays the negative effects of unchecked industrial processes on the ecosystem, serving as a commentary on the potential harm that can result from human actions. This ecological awareness aligns with the broader themes of environmental consciousness that can be found in some of Heaney's works.

The poem uses both cognitive and affective resonance to convey its themes and emotions. The sensory imagery and detailed descriptions of the flax cultivation process engage readers cognitively by allowing them to visualize and comprehend the industrial processes involved. The poem's depiction of the stages of cultivation, decay, and processing draws readers into the narrative, creating a cognitive connection with the subject matter. At the same time, the poem taps into affective resonance by evoking emotions associated with the consequences of the flax decay. The vivid descriptions of the foul odor, contamination, and impact on the environment elicit visceral reactions in readers. The juxtaposition of the natural world and the industrial process triggers emotions related to human impact on the environment and the consequences of human actions.

5.6 Sruth

The poem "Sruth," written by Seamus Heaney in memory of Mary O Muirithe, is part of his poetry collection "Electric Light," which was published in 2001. "Electric Light" is one of Heaney's later collections and continues his exploration of themes related to nature, memory, language, and human experiences. The collection showcases Heaney's skill in crafting evocative imagery and reflecting on personal and universal themes. Heaney uses the word "sruth" for its title. This lexeme does not appear in the OED because it is an Irish word that etymologically comes from Proto-Celtic srutom from Proto-Indo-European srew. Cognate with Welsh ffrdrwd and maybe the Gaulish hydronym Phroudis. It means "steam, current, flow and electricity." This is the poem:

> The bilingual race
> And truth of that water
> Spilling down Errigal,
>
> The sruth like the rush
> Of its downpour translated
> Into your accent:
>
> You in your dishabills
> Washing your face
> In the guttural glen.
>
> Mountain and maiden.
> The shard of a mirror.
> Your head in the air
>
> Of that childhood breac-Ghaeltacht,
> Those sky-maiden haunts
> You would tell me about
>
> Again and again-
> Then asked me to visit:
> If anything happened
>
> Just to see and be sure
> And not to forget
> For your sake to do it.
>
> Splash of clear water.
> Things out in the open.
> The spoken word, "cancer."

Textual Analysis

> And now it has happened
> I see what I saw
> On the morning you asked me:
>
> Neck-baring snowdrops-
> Like you at the sruth
> First-footing springtime,
>
> Fit for what comes.

Following the model of textual analysis provided in Section 4.1, we might highlight the following elements from this text:

1. Metaphoric Potential:
   - The imagery of "truth of that water/Spilling down Errigal" and "sruth like the rush/Of its downpour translated/Into your accent" combines natural elements with linguistic associations.
   - The metaphor of "truth of that water" implies authenticity and purity.
2. Synesthetic Potential:
   - The phrase "washing your face/In the guttural glen" combines visual and auditory sensations, creating a synesthetic experience.
3. Cognitive Blending:
   - Conceptual integration takes place in the lines "Mountain and maiden./The shard of a mirror./Your head in the air" blend nature ("Mountain"), human presence ("maiden"), and reflection ("shard of a mirror").
4. Emotional Resonance:
   - The poem carries an emotional weight, reflecting nostalgia, personal attachment, and the emotional impact of significant events.
5. Contextual Analysis:
   - The poem explores personal memories and connections, particularly around the concept of "sruth" (stream) and its cultural significance.

- The reference to "cancer" introduces vulnerability and mortality into the narrative.
- Mary, wife of Diarmaid Ó'Muirithe, distinguished Irish lexicographer and etymologist, was admired by Heaney for her courage facing death from cancer. In his childhood she was 4 years his senior in the breac-Gaeltacht camp. He sees her as a relevant figure in his life worth honoring.
6. Reader's Perspective:
    - Readers may interpret the poem through their own experiences with nature, memory, and emotional connections.
    - The theme of facing difficult news and memories resonates with individuals who have dealt with challenging circumstances.
7. Thematic Exploration:
    - The poem shows the intertwining of nature, language, memory, and emotional connections.
    - It suggests how personal experiences are intertwined with linguistic and cultural elements.

The poem navigates personal and emotional terrain using nature as a backdrop for deeper exploration. Through metaphoric potential, synesthetic qualities, cognitive blending, emotional resonance, context, reader perspectives, and thematic exploration, Heaney creates a multi-layered piece that invites readers to contemplate their own relationships and connections.

Heaney provides an evocative narrative that resonates with themes of memory, human connection, and the passage of time. While a poem and a short story are distinct literary forms, "Sruth" embodies certain elements of storytelling and conceptualization within its condensed structure:

- Narrative Essence: "Sruth" encapsulates a narrative essence by presenting a sequence of events and emotions that unfold in a chronological order. The poem begins with vivid imagery of water spilling down Errigal and progresses through the narrator's memories and experiences.

- Setting and Characters: The poem establishes a sense of setting through descriptions of landscapes, such as Errigal, and introduces characters like the narrator and the individual referred to in the poem.
- Emotional Journey: The poem captures an emotional journey—from childhood memories and shared experiences to facing the reality of difficult news.

The poem's imagery, such as "washing your face/In the guttural glen" and "neck-baring snowdrops" adds depth to the narrative and offers symbolic layers. Readers can empathize with the narrator's emotions and the themes explored in the poem. In essence, while "Sruth" is a poem, it encapsulates elements of narrative structure, character interactions, emotional arcs, and thematic exploration that echo the qualities of a short story. So, we can identify certain elements that could be seen as a beginning, middle, and end to provide a sense of progression:

- Beginning: The beginning of the poem introduces the concept of the "bilingual race" and the "truth of that water" spilling down Errigal. This sets the tone for the exploration of language, culture, and memory that follows.
- Middle: The middle section of the poem focuses on the speaker's memories and experiences related to the bilingual environment and the landscape. It describes the rush of the water, the speaker's connection to it, and the feeling of being translated into a different accent. This section shows the speaker's personal reflections on language and identity.
- End: The end of the poem shifts to a more introspective and contemplative tone. It references the idea of "first-footing springtime," suggesting a renewal or beginning. The speaker reflects on the significance of memories and experiences, as well as the importance of remembering and visiting places from the past. This ending section wraps up the themes of language, memory, and connection.

The poem's structure is more about creating an impression and conveying a particular atmosphere, rather than following a traditional narrative arc. Its thematic cohesion ties the various images together, providing a snapshot of the speaker's thoughts and memories related to a specific time and place. The poem invites readers to experience an emotional journey through condensed storytelling and prompts contemplation of personal memories, human connections, and the passage of time.

The vivid sensory imagery appeals to the reader's cognitive senses, allowing them to mentally visualize and immerse themselves in the scenes depicted in the poem. This cognitive engagement helps create a strong connection between the reader and the poem's content. Moreover, the poem's exploration of memory, language, and personal reflection triggers affective resonance by eliciting emotions and feelings in the reader. The emotional themes of identity, nostalgia, and connection to one's roots resonate with readers' own experiences and emotions, creating a sense of shared sentiment.

The interplay between cognitive engagement and affective resonance is what makes "Sruth" a powerful and impactful piece. By inviting readers to not only intellectually understand the poem but also emotionally connect with its themes, Heaney creates a holistic experience that lingers in the reader's mind and heart, fostering a deeper appreciation for the poem's complexity and depth.

5.7 Final Remarks

The analysis of these poems could not be completed without highlighting one remarkable element in Heaney's works, that is, the constant use of water or liquidity, often possessing a special iconic power due to its ability to evoke a range of emotions, sensations, and symbolic meanings.

Water's fluidity, transparency, and transformative nature make it a versatile symbol that can represent various aspects of human experience and the natural world. Often seen as a purifying force, water symbolizes renewal and fresh beginnings, washing away troubles and heralding personal growth. Its life-giving properties connect it to themes of purity, birth and fertility, embodying the essence of creation and nurturing. Water's fluidity aligns with emotions and the ever-shifting human experience, capturing feelings and the dynamic nature of existence.

Moreover, water's depths serve as a metaphor for the subconscious, representing hidden emotions and the mysteries lying beneath the surface. Its ability to transition and journey mirrors life's passages, signifying transformations and the challenges that accompany them. The adaptability seen in water's changing forms reflects the capacity to navigate change and adversity with flexibility. Evoking spiritual and mystical connotations, water bridges the material and spiritual realms, hinting at the divine and the transcendent.

Across Seamus Heaney's poetry, water's symbolism resonates deeply. The iconic power of water lies in its capacity to convey complex themes in a tangible and relatable way. In the context of the poems mentioned in this chapter we can see the following:

- In "The First Words," the iconic power of water lies in its metaphorical representation of change and contamination, which adds depth to the exploration of memory and language.
- In "Remembered Columns," water's iconic power may stem from its ability to symbolize memory's fluid nature and its interaction with solid pillars of tradition.
- In "Lint Water," water's iconic power is evident in its role as a symbol of pollution and decay caused by industrial processes, highlighting the impact of human actions on the environment.
- In "Sruth," water's iconic power embodies the flow of language, culture, and heritage, symbolizing the enduring connection between the speakers and their origins.

Water's versatility as a symbol allows it to resonate with readers on various levels, inviting them to engage emotionally, intellectually, and sensorially with the themes presented in Heaney's poetry. And it resonates even more in each one of us when we get to know that, just ten days before dying, Heaney submitted a poem for a new collection, published with the participation of more than fifty other writers later, in 2014 (Flood, 2014). For that he chose carefully to elevate water to the status of person, putting literal words in its mouth as follows:

> Water says, 'My place here is in dream,
> In quiet good standing. Like a sleeping stream,
> Come rain or sullen shine I'm peaceable.'
> ("Gustave Caillebotte, c.1872." Lines 6–8)

This lyrical personification imbues water with a voice and consciousness, underscoring Heaney's inclination for breathing life into the elements of his poetry. It reinforces the complex relationship between humans and nature, and how even in his final days, Heaney found creative solace and connection through his enduring poetic exploration of the world around him.

Finally, to wrap up this chapter, we will travel succinctly through the common elements and themes that emerged from the four poems analyzed under our textual analysis model (see Sections 4.2, 4.3, 4.4 and 4.5):

1. Nature and Environment: All four poems incorporate vivid descriptions of nature and the environment, whether it is the "water honeyed in the slung bucket" in "The First Words," the "remembered columns" in "Remembered Columns," the process of flax processing and the concept of water in "Lint Water," or the imagery of water and landscapes in "Sruth."
2. Emotional Resonance: Each poem carries emotional weight and invites readers to connect on a personal and emotional level. Whether it is the nostalgic memories in "The First Words," the reflection on the past in "Remembered Columns," the poignant imagery in "Lint Water," or the emotional journey of "Sruth," all poems evoke emotions and memories.
3. Cultural and Linguistic Elements: The poems exhibit a strong connection to cultural and linguistic elements. Whether it is the bilingual race and linguistic influences in "The First Words," the idea of remembered columns as linguistic remnants in "Remembered Columns," the mention of "Lint water" as a cultural

practice in "Lint Water," or the concept of "sruth" (stream) and linguistic connections in "Sruth," language and culture play integral roles.
4. Narrative and Storytelling: While these are poems, they embody narrative qualities. They present sequences of events, emotions, and experiences that resonate with elements of storytelling. This is seen in the progression of memories in "The First Words," the reminiscence of past events in "Remembered Columns," the process of flax processing and its consequences in "Lint Water," and the emotional journey in "Sruth."
5. Human Connection and Interaction: The poems involve interactions and connections between individuals, whether it is the speaker addressing someone in "The First Words," the contemplation of a figure from the past in "Remembered Columns," the emotional connection to a person or a place in "Lint Water," or the bond between the narrator and the person addressed in "Sruth."
6. Reflection on Time: All four poems reflect on the passage of time, whether through memories, the impact of past events, or the changes in environments over time.
7. Imagery and Sensory Experience: Each poem employs rich imagery and sensory details to evoke emotions and immerse readers in the scenes. Whether it is the visual and auditory elements in "The First Words," the metaphorical and reflective imagery in "Remembered Columns," the sensory experiences in "Lint Water," or the combination of nature and memories in "Sruth," imagery is a consistent feature.

In conclusion, these poems by Seamus Heaney, randomly selected, share commonalities in their focus on nature, emotional resonance, cultural and linguistic aspects, narrative qualities, human connections, reflection on time, and vivid imagery. These themes collectively contribute to Heaney's exploration of memory, emotion, and human experience through his distinctive poetic voice.

CHAPTER 6

Conclusions

Short story is not merely a component of literature but also an essential cognitive capacity inherent to human thinking, capable of making meaning iconic when it stands for an idea or a cluster of ideas that are widely recognized and emotionally or culturally significant. Everyday narratives assist us in comprehending reality, revealing how our experiences, knowledge, and thoughts are structured. This helps cognitive scientists in deciphering human cognition and the workings of the mind. However, Cognitive Studies bring a fresh perspective to the realm of short story analysis. They introduce novel inquiries, such as what prompts us to employ stories for thinking, recalling, and remembering? How does the human mind exhibit remarkable creativity in using narratives? Why is storytelling deeply embedded within the mechanisms of the mind? Why do stories frequently impart guidance on how to live and what to value?

Furthermore, the overarching schema of a story significantly influences how individuals recall information freely, impacting the recollection of both specific details and the story's essence. This schema's influence on memory organization endures over time, reinforcing the more abstract and universal elements of the narrative (Yussen et al., 1988). In a general context, some scholars propose that in human development, "event memory" emerges earlier, while "narrativity" develops later (Lounsberry et al., 1998: 148). However, separating an event from its temporal, spatial, authoritative, causal, and goal-oriented aspects, presents a challenge. These elements, even if not consciously recognized or explicitly identified, are integral to a story and must be present. They require inclusion and re-indexing within our human framework for comprehending reality. Therefore, the story is foundational and elemental, representing the convergence of event memory and narrativity processes.

The iconic power of the short story lies in its remarkable ability to encapsulate the essence of human experiences and emotions within a condensed form, intertwining meaning and narrative compactly. Drawing a parallel to a masterful painting that captures the depth of a scene using minimal brushstrokes, the short story uses brevity as its canvas to conjure vibrant imagery, provoke contemplation, and evoke profound sentiments. This unique potency stems from the efficiency of language, enabling writers to distill complicated themes, characters, and situations into a concise narrative that resonates deeply with readers.

In turn, the short story's capacity to evoke both cognitive understanding and emotional engagement elevates it as a powerful instrument for diving into cultural intricacies, cognitive processes, and human connections. This potency is greatly illustrated in the literary works of Seamus Heaney. The poems chosen for textual analysis, including "The Haw Lantern," "The First Words," "Remembered Columns," "Lint Water," and "Sruth," exhibit an iconic power harnessed through a synergy of language, imagery, and thematic exploration. Each poem resonates with readers on multiple levels:

1. "The Haw Lantern": The iconic power of this poem emerges from its use of metaphor and symbolism surrounding the image of the lantern. It explores themes of enlightenment and the search for moral guidance in darkness, effectively weaving together personal introspection with broader philosophical queries.
2. "The First Words": This poem's iconic power lies in its evocation of bilingualism, memory, and connection. It captures the essence of language's role in bridging cultures while diving into personal memory's depth and the emotional significance attached to initial words.
3. "Remembered Columns": The iconic power of this poem is manifest in the metaphor of columns as linguistic remnants and memories. These columns serve as literal and figurative pillars upholding the past, allowing readers to contemplate the interplay between spoken and written words and the enduring nature of memory.
4. "Lint Water": The poem "Lint Water" derives its iconic power from its vivid imagery of the flax-processing process, seamlessly

merging nature and human industry. The poem's language evokes sensory experiences, enabling readers to connect with the sights, scents, and emotions linked to this practice. The mention of "lint water" serves as a symbolic anchor for cultural practices and their significance.
5. "Sruth": The iconic power of "Sruth" resides in its capacity to traverse time and invoke emotions through nature and personal connection. The imagery of water and landscapes becomes a conduit for exploring memory, relationships, and addressing challenging news, imparting the poem with a timeless and resonant quality.

Across these poems we can see how the iconic power stems from Heaney's mastery of language, his skillful use of imagery, and his ability to condense complex themes into succinct and evocative verses. The poems tap into the human experience—whether through linguistic connections, memory, cultural practices, or emotional landscapes—and invite readers to reflect, empathize, and connect with the universal themes they explore.

This iconic power is further elevated by Heaney's refined application of synesthesia, a cognitive device interweaving sensory experiences to evoke heightened emotional and imaginative responses. Synesthetic elements enhance the poems' iconic power by invoking multisensory engagement, connecting language and emotion on a profound level. Whether it is the "water honeyed" in "The First Words," the "remembered columns" in "Remembered Columns," the tactile and olfactory sensations of "Lint Water," or the imagery of "washing your face" in "Sruth," these elements enrich the poems' resonance by fostering a deeper connection between language and emotion.

In essence, Seamus Heaney, the "poet of the senses," orchestrates a symphony where the iconic power of the short story and poetry seamlessly intertwines culture, cognition, and affective involvement. Through meticulous craftsmanship, Heaney invites readers to embark on journeys of thought and emotion, using cognitive tools like metaphor, synesthesia, and blending. By doing so, he demonstrates the profound bond between storytelling, cognition, and cultural resonance, leaving an indelible mark through the enduring impact of his work.

Bibliography

Anderson, Richard C. "Inferences about the World Meanings," in Arthur C. Graesser and Gordon H. Bower (eds.), *Inferences and Text Comprehension*. New York: Academic Press, 1987, pp. 1–16.

Andrews, Elmer. *Seamus Heaney: A Collection of Critical Essays*. Berlin: Springer, 1992.

Barcelona, Antonio. *Metaphor and Metonymy at the Crossroads*. Berlin: De Gruyter, 2000.

Barsalou, Lawrence W. "Perceptual Symbol Systems," *Behavioral and Brain Sciences*, Vol. 22, no. 3, 1999, pp. 577–609.

Barsalou, Lawrence W. "Grounded Cognition," *Annual Review Psychology*, Vol. 59, 2008, pp. 617–645.

Barsalou, Lawrence W. (2020). "Challenges and Opportunities for Grounding Cognition," *Journal of Cognition*, Vol.3, no. 1, 2020, pp. 1–24. DOI: <https://doi.org/10.5334/joc.116>.

Bloom, Harold. *The Anxiety of Influence: A Theory of Poetry*. Oxford: Oxford University Press, 1997.

Boroditsky, Lera. "Metaphoric Structuring: Understanding Time through Spatial Metaphors," *Cognition*, Vol. 75, 2000, pp. 1–28.

Boroditsky, Lera. "How Language Shapes Thought," *Scientific American*, Vol. 304, no. 2, 2011, pp. 62–65.

Bretones Callejas, Carmen M. "Synaesthetic Metaphors in English," *ICSI Technical Reports*. 2001, <http://www.icsi.berkeley.edu/ftp/pub/techreports/2001/tr-01-008.pdf>

Bretones Callejas, Carmen M. "Entrevista a Charles J. Fillmore," *ODISEA. Revista de estudios ingleses*, Vol. 4, 2003, pp. 41–48.

Bretones Callejas, Carmen M. "Synesthesia," in Keith Brown and Ronald E. Asher (eds.), *Encyclopedia of Language and Linguistics*. Amsterdam: Elsevier, 2005, pp. 367–370.

Bretones Callejas, Carmen M. "Enfoque cognitivo para el desarrollo de políticas de interculturalidad en el aula de estudios ingleses," in Carmen-Cayetana Castro Moreno (ed.), *Facetas multiculturales en producción y traducción: Metáforas, alegorías y otras imágenes*. Granada: Comares, 2020, pp. 329–336.

Bretones Callejas, Carmen M. "La imaginación como capacidad cognitiva indispensable," in Josefina Rodriguez Góngora et al. *Psicología Siglo XXI: Una mirada amplia e integrad*a. Madrid: Dykinson, 2022, pp. 425–442.

Bretones Callejas, Carmen M. and Chamizo-Domínguez, Pedro J. "Euphemisms, Proverbs, Allusions, and Cognition: A Study of Two Poems by Antonio Machado," *Círculo de lingüística aplicada a la comuniciación*, Vol. 22, 2005, pp. 1–16.

Bretones Callejas, Carmen M., Ridao Rodrigo, Susana and Alarcón Hermosilla, Salvador. "Language, Cognition and Style: An Introduction to the Cognitive Stylistics Section," *Odisea*, Vol. 22, 2021, pp. 9–13.

Brosch, Renate. "Reading and Visualisation," *Anglistik*, Vol. 24, no. 2, 2013, pp. 169–179.

Brosch, Renate. "Experiencing Short Stories: A Cognitive Approach Focusing on Reading Narrative Space," in Jochen Achilles and Ina Bergmann (eds.), *Liminality and the Short Story*. New York: Routledge, 2014, pp. 92–107.

Brosch, Renate. "18. Images in Narrative Literature: Cognitive Experience and Iconic Moments". In Gabriele Rippl (ed.), *Handbook of Intermediality*: Literature - Image - Sound - Music, Berlin, München, Boston: De Gruyter, 2015, pp. 343-360. https://doi.org/10.1515/9783110311075-020.

Brosch, Renate. "The Iconic Power of Short Stories – A Cognitive Approach". In Ronja Bodola and Guido Isekenmeier (eds.), *Literary Visualities: Visual Descriptions, Readerly Visualisations, Textual Visibilities*, Berlin: De Gruyter, 2017, pp. 165-200. https://doi.org/10.1515/9783110378030-006.

Brosch, Renate. "What We 'see' When We Read: Visualization and Vividness in Reading Fictional Narratives," *Cortex*, Vol. 105, 2018a, pp. 135–143 DOI: 10.1016/j.cortex.2017.08.020.

Brosch, Renate. "Ekphrasis in the Digital Age: Responses to Image," *Poetics Today*, Vol. 39, no. 2, 2018b, pp. 225–243 https://doi.org/10.1215/03335372-4324420.

Brown, Calvin S. *Music and Literature: A Comparison of the Arts*. University Press of New England, 1989.

Cacciari, Cristina. "Why Do We Speak Metaphorically? Reflections on the Functions of Metaphor in Discourse and Reasoning," in Albert N. Katz, Cristina Cacciari, Raymond W. Gibbs, Jr., and Mark Turner (eds.), *Figurative Language and Thought*. New York: Oxford University Press, 1998, pp. 119–157.

Cacciari, Cristina. "The place of idioms in a literal and metaphorical world," in Christina Cacciari and Patricia Tabossi (eds.), *Idioms: Processing, structure, and interpretation*. Mahwah, New Jersey: Lawrence Erlbaum Associates. 1999, pp. 27–55.

Clark, Herbert H. *Arenas of Language Use.* Chicago: University of Chicago Press, 1992.
Corcoran, N. (1986). Seamus Heaney. London: Faber and Faber.
Corcoran, N. (2014). *Poetry & Responsibility.* Vol. 6. Oxford University Press.
Corcoran, N., & Heaney, S. (1998). *A Critical Study.* Vol. 236. London: faber and faber.
Cortés de los Ríos, M. Enriqueta and Bretones Callejas, Carmen M. "Estudio cognitivo del componente visual en la publicidad de automóviles," in Mary Frances Litzler, Jesús García Laborda and Cristina Tejedor Martínez (eds), *Beyond the Universe of Languages for Specific Purposes: The 21st Century Perspective,* 2016, pp. 171–180.
Curtis, Tony. *The Art of Seamus Heaney.* Dublin: Wolfhound Press, 1985.
Crystal, David. *The English Language.* London: Penguin Books, 1988.
Cytowic, Richard E. "Synesthesia: Phenomenology and Neuropsychology: A Review of Current Knowledge," *PSYCHE,* Vol. 2, no. 10, 1995 pp. 2–10.
Cytowic, Richard E. *The Man Who Tasted Shapes.* Cambridge, Massachusetts MIT Press, 2003.
Cytowic, Richard E. *The Stone Age Brain in the Screen Age.* Cambridge, Massachusetts MIT Press, 2024.
Damasio, Antonio. *Feeling and Knowing: Making Minds Conscious.* New York: Pantheon Books Pantheon, 2021.
Eliot, T. S. "Tradition and the Individual Talent," *The Egoist,* Vol. 7, no. 2, 1920, pp. 62–64.
Fauconnier, Giles and Turner, Mark. "Blending as a Central Process of Grammar," in Adele Goldberg (ed.), *Conceptual Structure, Discourse, and Language.* Stanford: Center for the Study of Language and Information, 1996, pp. 113–129.
Fauconnier, Gilles and Turner, Mark. *The Way We Think: Conceptual Blending and the Mind's Hidden Complexities.* London: Basic Books, 2002.
Fennell, Desmond. *Whatever You Say, Say Nothing: Why Seamus Heaney Is No. 1.* Dublin: ELO Publications, 1991.
Fillmore, Charles J. "An Alternative to Checklist Theories of Meaning," *Proceedings of the Berkeley Linguistics Society,* Vol. 1, 1975, pp. 123–131.
Fillmore, Charles J. "Frame Semantics," in Linguistic Society of Korea (ed.), *Linguistics in the Morning Calm.* Hanshin: Linguistic Society of Korea Seoul, 1982, pp. 111–138.
Fillmore, Charles J. "Frame Semantics," in Dirk Geeraerts (ed.), *Cognitive Linguistics: Basic Readings.* Amsterdam: Mouton de Gruyter, 2006, pp. 373–400.
Fillmore, Charles J. "Border Conflicts: FrameNet meets Construction Grammar," in Elisenda Bernal and Janet DeCesaris (eds.), *Proceedings of the XIII EURALEX*

International Congress (Barcelona, 15–19 July 2008), Barcelona: Pompeu Fabra. 2008, pp. 49–68.

Fillmore, Charles J. "Berkeley Construction Grammar," in Thomas Hoffmann and Graeme Trousdale (eds.), *The Oxford Handbook on Construction Grammar*. Oxford: Oxford University Press, 2013, pp. 111–132.

Flood, Alison. "Seamus Heaney's Last Poem Published in Irish Gallery's Anthology," *The Guardian*, 2014, October 3, Belfast, https://www.theguardian.com/books/2014/oct/03/seamus-heaney-last-poem-national-gallery-ireland-anthology

Freeman, Margaret H. "Cognitive Linguistic Approaches to Literary Studies: State of the Art in Cognitive Poetics," in Thomas Hoffmann and Graeme Trousdale (eds.), *The Oxford Handbook on Cognitive Linguistics*. Oxford: Oxford University Press, 2010, pp. 1175–1202.

Freeman, Margaret H. "Poetry and the Scope of Metaphor: Toward a Cognitive Theory of Literature," in Antonio Barcelona (ed.), *Metaphor and Metonymy at the Crossroads: A Cognitive Perspective*. Berlin: Mouton de Gruyter, 2012, pp. 253–282.

Gallese, Vitorio and Lakoff, George. "The Brain's Concepts: The Role of the Sensory-motor System in Reason and Language," *Cognitive Neuropsychology*, Vol. 22, 2005, pp. 455–479.

Geeraerts, Dirk, and Hubert Cuyckens (eds.), *The Oxford Handbook of Cognitive Linguistics*, Oxford Handbooks (2010; online edn, Oxford Academic, 18 Sept. 2012), https://doi.org/10.1093/oxfordhb/9780199738632.001.0001.

Gibbs, Raymond W. *The Poetics of Mind: Figurative Thought, Language and Understanding*. Cambridge: Cambridge University Press, 1994.

Gibbs, Raymond W. "Taking Metaphor Out of Our Heads and Putting It into the Cultural World," in Raymond W. Gibbs and Gerard Steen (eds.), *Metaphor in Cognitive Linguistics*. Amsterdam: John Benjamins, 1999, pp. 146–166.

Goldberg, Adele. *Constructions: A Construction Grammar Approach to Argument Structure*. Chicago: The University of Chicago Press, 1995.

Grady, Joseph E. "Theories Are Buildings Revisited," *Cognitive Linguistics*, Vol. 8, no. 4, 1997, pp. 267–290.

Grady, Joseph E. "Image Schemas and Perception: Refining a Definition," in *From Perception to Meaning*. Beate Hampe, Berlin: Mouton de Gruyter. 2005, pp. 35–55.

Grady, Joseph E., Oakley, Todd, and Coulson, Seana. "Blending and Metaphor," in G. Steen and R. Gibbs (eds.), *Metaphor in Cognitive Linguistics*. Philadelphia: John Benjamins, 1999.

Graesser, Arthur C., Millis, Keith M., and Zwaan, Rolf A. "Discourse Comprehension," *Annual Review of Psychology*, Vol. 48, 1997, pp. 163–189.

Bibliography

Guerra, Juani. "Short Story and Cognition: Effects in Literary Studies and in the Socio-cultural Evolution of a Robust Narrative Genre," in Maurice A. Lee and Aaron Penn (eds.), *Beyond History: The Radiance of the Short Story*. Philadelphia Lee and Penn Publishing, 2019, pp. 4–13.

Ibáñez Ibáñez, José R, Fernández Sánchez, José F., and Bretones Callejas, Carmen M. (2007). *Contemporary Debates on the Short Story*. Bern: Peter Lang.

Hart, Henry. *Seamus Heaney: Poet of Contrary Progressions*. Syracuse, NY: Syracuse University Press, 1992.

Heaney, Seamus. *Death of a Naturalist*. London: Faber and Faber, 1966.

Heaney, Seamus. *Wintering Out*. London: Faber and Faber, 1972.

Heaney, Seamus. *Preoccupations: Selected Prose, 1968–1978*. New York: Farrar, Straus and Giroux, 1980.

Heaney, Seamus. *The Haw Lantern*. New York: The Noonday Press, 1987.

Heaney, Seamus. *The Government of Tongue: The 1986 T. S. Eliot Memorial Lectures and Other Critical Writings*. London: Faber and Faber, 1988.

Heaney, Seamus. *The Spirit Level*. London: Faber & Faber, 1995.

Heaney, Seamus. *Diary of the One Who Vanished*. London: Faber and Faber, 1999.

Heaney, Seamus. *Finders Keepers: Selected Prose 1971–2001*. New York: Farrar Straus & Giroux, 2002.

Heaney, Seamus. *District and Circle*. London: Faber and Faber, 2006.

Heaney, Seamus. *Human Chain*. London: Faber and Faber, 2010.

Herman, David. *Story Logic: Problems and Possibilities of Narrative*. University of Nebraska Press, 2002.

Herman, David. *Narrative Theory and the Cognitive Sciences*. Chicago: Chicago University Press, 2003.

Herman, David. "Quantitative Methods in Narratology: A Corpus-based Study of Motion Event in Stories," in Jan Christoph Meister (ed.), *Narratology Beyond Literary Criticism: Mediality, Disciplinarity*. Berlin: De Gruyter, 2005, pp. 125–149.

Herman, David. "Storytelling and the Sciences of Mind: Cognitive Narratology, Discursive Psychology, and Narratives in Face-to-face Interaction," *Narrative*, Vol. 15, 2007, pp. 306–334.

Herman, David. "Cognitive Narratology," *Handbook of Narratology*, Vol. 1, 2009, pp. 30–43.

Herman, David. *Storytelling and the Sciences of Mind*. Cambridge, Massachusetts: MIT Press, 2013.

Higgins, Geraldin. "Introduction," in Geraldine Higgins (ed.), *Seamus Heaney in Context*. Cambridge: Cambridge University Press, 2021, pp. 1–12.

Hughes, Brian. *Antología Poética de Seamus Heaney*. Diputación de Alicante. Instituto de Cultura Juan Gil-Albert, 1993.

Hurlburt, George F. and Voas, Jeffrey. "Storytelling: From Cave Art to Digital Media," *IT Professional*, Vol. 13, no. 5, 2011, pp. 4–7.
Ibáñez-Ibáñez, José Ramón, Fernández Sánchez, José Francisco, and Bretones Callejas, Carmen M. *Contemporary Debates on the Short Story*. Bern: Peter Lang, 2007.
Ibaretxe-Antuñano, Iraide. "Metaphorical Mappings in the Sense of Smell," in Raymond Gibbs and Gerard Steen (eds.), *Metaphor in Cognition*. Amsterdam: John Benjamins, 1999, pp. 29–45.
Johnson, Mark. *The Body in the Mind*. Chicago: Chicago University Press, 1987.
Kiberd, Declan. *The Irish Writer and the World*. Cambridge: Cambridge University Press, 2005.
Kövecses, Zoltan. *Metaphor and Emotion*. Cambridge: Cambridge University Press, 2000.
Kövecses, Zoltan. "Perception and Metaphor," *Perception Metaphors*, Vol. 19, no. 327, 2019, pp. 10–75.
Lakoff, George. *Women, Fire, and Dangerous Things*. Chicago: University of Chicago Press, 1987.
Lakoff, George. "Explaining Embodied Cognition Results," *Topics in Cognitive Science*, Vol. 4, no. 4, 2012, pp. 773–785.
Lakoff, George, and Johnson, Mark. *Metaphors We Live By*. Chicago: University of Chicago Press, 1980.
Lakoff, George, and Johnson, Mark. *Philosophy in the Flesh*. New York: Basic Books, 1999.
Lakoff, George, and Turner, Mark. *More Than Cool Reason: A Field Guide to Poetic Metaphor*. Chicago: University of Chicago Press, 1989.
Langacker, Ronald. *Foundations of Cognitive Grammar*. Stanford: Stanford University Press, 1987.
Lewis, Clive S. *On Stories and Other Essays on Literature*. Orlando: Harvest, 1982.
Lewis, Clive S. *Image and Imagination: Essays and Reviews*. In Walter Hooper (ed.). New York: Cambridge University Press., 2013.
Lohafer, Susan, and Lohafer, Susan. *Reading for Storyness: Preclosure Theory, Empirical Poetics, and Culture in the Short Story*. Baltimore: Johns Hopkins University Press, 2003.
Longley, Edna. *The Living Stream: Literature & Revisionism in Ireland*. Newcastle: Bloodaxe Books, 1994.
Lounsberry, Barbara, Feddersen, Rick, Lohafer, Susan, and Rohrberger, Mary. *The Tales We Tell: Perspectives on the Short Story*. Westport, Praeger, 1998.
Mars-Jones, Adam. "Gimmicky Amis Not at His Best," *Mail & Guardian*, January 8, 1999.

Marvell, Andrew. *The Garden*. Poetry Foundation. From https://www.poetryfoundation.org/poems/44682/the-garden-56d223dec2ced [Accessed March 5, 2021].

May, Charles. *The Short Story: The Reality of Artifice*. New York: Routledge, 2013.

Miall, David S., and Kuiken, Don. "A Feeling for Fiction: Becoming What We Behold," *Poetics*, Vol. 30, no. 4, 2002, pp. 221–241.

Neil, Corcoran. *The Poetry of Seamus Heaney: A Critical Study*. London: Faber and Faber, 1998.

Oatley, Keith. "Fiction: Simulation of Social Worlds," *Trends in Cognitive Sciences*, Vol. 20, no. 8, 2016, pp. 618–628.

O'Brien, Eugene. *Seamus Heaney and the Place of Writing*. Gainesville, FL: University Press of Florida, 2002.

O'Donoghue, Bernard. *Seamus Heaney and the Language of Poetry*. Routledge, 2017.

Oxford English Dictionary (OED). Oxford: Oxford University Press. <https://www.oed.com>.

Parini, Jay. "The Bog Poet," *The Nation*, January 4, 1999.

Parker, Michael. *Seamus Heaney: The Making of the Poet*. Iowa: University of Iowa Press, 1993.

Peña-Cervel, María Sandra, and de Mendoza Ibáñez, Francisco José Ruiz. *Figuring Out Figuration: A Cognitive Linguistic Account*. Amsterdam: John Benjamins, 2022.

Pereira, Margarida E. "Stories within Stories: Fairy Tales as Intertextual Fragments in AS Byatt's Possession: A Romance," in Maurice A. Lee and Aaron Penn (eds.), *Beyond History: The Radiance of the Short Story*. Philadelphia: Lee and Penn Publishing, 2019, pp. 181–192.

Perloff, Marjorie. *Unoriginal Genius: Poetry by Other Means in the New Century*. Chicago: University of Chicago Press, 2010.

Prinz, Jesse J. "Is Emotion a Form of Perception?," *Canadian Journal of Philosophy*, Vol. 36, supplement Vol. 32, 2006, pp. 137–160.

Roberts, Brady R. T., MacLeod, Colin M., and Fernandes, Myra A. "Symbol Superiority: Why $ Is Better Remembered Than 'dollar,'" *Cognition*, Vol. 238, 2023, p. 105435.

Rohrer, Tim. "The Cognitive Science of Metaphor from Philosophy to Neuropsychology," *Theoria et Historia Scientiarum*, Vol. 6, no. 1, 2002, pp. 27–42.

Rollins, Hyder Edward. *The Letters of John Keats: Volume 1, 1814–1818*. Cambridge: Cambridge University Press, 2012, pp. 80–85.

Rosch, Eleonor. *Principles of Categorization: Cognition and Categorization*. Hillsdale, NJ: Lawrence Erlbaum, 1978, pp. 27–48.

Sachs, Matthew E., Ellis, Robert J., Schlaug, Gottfried and Loui, Psyche. "Brain Connectivity Reflects Human Aesthetic Responses to Music," *Social Cognitive and Affective Neuroscience*, Vol. 11, no. 6, 2016, pp. 884–891.
Schmidt, Michael. *Reading Modern Poetry*. London: Routledge, 1989.
Shen, Yeshayahu. "Cognitive Constrains on Poetic Figures," *Cognitive Linguistics*, Vol. 8, no. 1, 1997, pp. 33–71.
Sinha, Christopher. "Language as a Biocultural Niche and Social Institution," in Vyvyan Evans and Stéphanie Pourcel (eds.), *New Directions in Cognitive Linguistics*. Amsterdam: John Benjamins, 2009, pp. 289–310.
Sinha, Christopher. "Language and Other Artifacts: Socio-cultural Dynamics of Niche Construction," *Frontiers in Psychology*, Vol. 6, 2015, p. 1601.
Slobin, Dan I. "The Many Ways to Search for a Frog: Linguistic Typology and the Expression of Motion Events," in Ludo Verhoeven and Sven Stromqvist (eds.), *Relating Events in Narrative*, Vol. 2. London: Psychology Press, 2004, pp. 219–257.
Sontag, Susan. *On Photography*. New York: Farrar, Straus, and Giroux, 1977.
Soriano, Cristina. "Emotion and Conceptual Metaphor," in Helena Flam and Jochen Kleres (eds.), *Methods of Exploring Emotions*. London: Routledge, 2015, pp. 206–214.
Stansfield, John, and Bunce, Louise. "The Relationship between Empathy and Reading Fiction: Separate Roles for Cognitive and Affective Components," *Journal of European Psychology Students*, Vol. 5, no. 3, 2014, pp. 9–18.
Talmy, Leonard. *Toward a Cognitive Semantics. Volume I: Concept Structuring Systems*. Cambridge, MA: The Massachusetts Institute of Technology Press, 2000.
Talmy, Leonard. "The Representation of Spatial Structure in Spoken and Signed Language: A Neural Model," *Language and Linguistics*, Vol. 4, 2003, pp. 207–250.
Tomasello, Michael. *The Origins of Human Communication*. Cambridge, MA: MIT Press, 2008.
Toolan, Michael. "Engagement Via Emotional Heightening in "Passion": On the Grammatical Texture of Emotionally-immersive Passages in Short Fiction," *Narrative*, Vol. 20, no. 2, 2012, pp. 210–225.
Tsur, Reuven. *Toward a Theory of Cognitive Poetics*. Amsterdam: North-Holland, 1992.
Turner, Mark. *Reading Minds*. Princeton: Princeton University Press, 1991.
Turner, Mark. *The Literary Mind*. Oxford: Oxford University Press, 1996.
Turner, Mark. "Figure," in Albert N. Katz (ed.), *Figurative Language and Thought*. Oxford: Oxford University Press, 1998, pp. 44–87.
Turner, Mark, and Faucconier, Gilles. "A Conceptual Integration and Formal Expression," *Journal of Metaphor and Symbolic Activity*, Vol. 10, no. 3, 1995, pp. 183–204.

Turner, Mark, and Faucconier, Gilles. "A Mechanism of Creativity," *Poetics Today*, Vol. 20, no. 3, 1997, pp. 397–418.
Ullmann, Stephen. *Language and Style*. Oxford: Basil Blackwell, 1964.
Vendler, Helen. "Seamus Heaney." In Roger Matuz (ed.), *Contemporary Literary Criticism*, vol. 74, Detroit: Gale Research, 1992, pp. 149–200.
Vendler, Helen. *The Breaking of Style: Hopkins, Heaney, Graham*. Chicago: University of Chicago Press, 1995.
Vendler, Helen. *Seamus Heaney*. Cambridge: Harvard University Press, 1998.
Williams, Joseph M. "Synaesthetic Adjectives: A Possible Law of Semantic Change," *Language*, Vol. 52, no. 2, 1976, pp. 461–478.
Yussen, Steven, Huang, Shih-tseng, Mathews, Samuel, and Evans, Robert. "The Robustness and Temporal Course of the Story's Schema's Influence on Recall," *Journal of Experimental Psychology: Learning, Memory and Cognition*, Vol. 14, no. 1, 1988, pp. 173–179.
Zunshine, Lisa. *The Oxford Handbook of Cognitive Literary Studies*. Oxford: Oxford Handbooks, 2015.
Zwaan, Rolf A., Magliano, Joseph P., and Graesser, Arthur C. "Dimensions of Situation Model Construction in Narrative Comprehension," *Journal of Experimental Psychology: Learning, Memory and Cognition*, Vol. 21, 1995, pp. 162–197.

Annexe

Poems Used as Corpus of Investigation (Random Selection)

1. Death of a Naturalist (1966)
   1.1. Digging
   1.2. Death of a Naturalist
   1.3. Lint Water
   1.4. Personal Helicon
2. Door into the Dark (1969)
   2.1. The Peninsula
   2.2. The Wife's Tale
   2.3. Relic of Memory
   2.4. Bogland
   2.5. The Forge
   2.6. Requiem for the Croppies
3. Wintering Out (1972)
   3.1. Anahorish
   3.2. The other side
   3.3. Westering
4. Stations (1975)
   4.1. England's Difficulty
   4.2. Visitant
   4.3. The Stations of the West
5. North (1975)
   5.1. Mossbown
      I. Sunlight
      II. The Seed Cutters
   5.2. North
   5.3. Whatever You Say, Say Nothing
   5.4. Summer 1969

6. Field Work (1979)
    6.1. A Drink of Water
    6.2. An Afterwards
    6.3. A dream of Jealousy
7. Sweeney Astray (1983)
    7.1. Sweeney Astray
    7.2. Sweeney's Last Poem
8. Station Island (1984)
    8.1. The First Kingdom
    8.2. An Artist
    8.3. In Illo Tempore
    8.4. Away from it All
    8.5. The Underground
9. The Haw Lantern (1987)
    9.1. Form the Frontier of Writing
    9.2. From the Republic of Conscience
    9.3. From the Canton of Expectation
    9.4. From the Land of the Unspoken.
    9.5. The Haw Lantern.
10. The Spirit Level (1996)
    10.1. The Stick Rain
    10.2. To a Dutch Potter in Ireland
    10.3. Mint
    10.4. A Sofa in the Forties
    10.5. The Flight Path
    10.6. The First Words
    10.7. Remembered Columns
    10.8. Clearances - 3
    10.9. Clearances - 5
    10.10. Lightenings
        I.
        VI.
        VII.
        VIII.

11. Diary of One Who Vanished (1999)
    11.1. I
    11.2. XIV
    11.3. XV
    11.4. XVII
12. Electric Light (2001)
    12.1. At Toomebridge
    12.2. Perch
    12.3. Lupins
    12.4. Out of the Bag
    12.5. The Little Canticles of Asturias
    12.6. Red, White and Blue
        1. Red
        2. White
        3. Blue
    12.7. Vitruviana
    12.8. The Fragment
    12.9. On His Work in the English Tongue
    12.10. To the Shade of Zbigniew Herbert
    12.11. Arion
    12.12. Sruth
    12.13. Electric Light
13. District and Circle (2006)
    13.1. District and Circle
14. Human Chain (2010)
    14.1. Lick the Pencil
15. Posthumous Poem (Finished ten days before his death and published in a collective work in 2014)
    15.1. Gustave Caillebotte, c.1872

www.ingramcontent.com/pod-product-compliance
Ingram Content Group UK Ltd.
Pitfield, Milton Keynes, MK11 3LW, UK
UKHW022240230426
12048UKWH00018BA/1368